Nothing But Nets

Nothing But Nets

A Biography of Global Health Science
and Its Objects

Kirsten Moore-Sheeley

JOHNS HOPKINS UNIVERSITY PRESS   BALTIMORE

© 2023 Johns Hopkins University Press
All rights reserved. Published 2023
Printed in the United States of America on acid-free paper
9 8 7 6 5 4 3 2 1

Johns Hopkins University Press
2715 North Charles Street
Baltimore, Maryland 21218
www.press.jhu.edu

Library of Congress Cataloging-in-Publication Data is available.

ISBN 978-1-4214-4757-5 (hardcover)
ISBN 978-1-4214-4758-2 (ebook)

A catalog record for this book is available from the British Library.

Special discounts are available for bulk purchases of this book. For more information, please contact Special Sales at specialsales@jh.edu.

For Austin
and for my parents, Janet and Ron Moore

Contents

Abbreviations

CDC	Centers for Disease Control and Prevention (United States)
DANIDA	Danish International Development Agency
DDT	dichlorodiphenyltrichloroethane
DFID	Department for International Development (United Kingdom)
EARN	Eastern Africa Roll Back Malaria Network
FIELDMAL	Applied Field Research in Malaria
GFATM	Global Fund to Fight AIDS, Tuberculosis and Malaria
GOK	Government of Kenya
IMF	International Monetary Fund
ITN	insecticide-treated net
KEMRI	Kenya Medical Research Institute
KSH	Kenyan shilling
LSHTM	London School of Hygiene and Tropical Medicine
MACEPA	Malaria Control and Elimination Partnership
MDG	Millennium Development Goal
MRC	Medical Research Council
NATNETS	National Insecticide Treated Nets Programme (Tanzania)
NGO	nongovernmental organization
PATH	Program for Appropriate Technology in Health
PBO	piperonyl butoxide
PMI	President's Malaria Initiative
PSI	Population Services International
RBM	Roll Back Malaria
TDR	Special Programme for Research and Training in Tropical Diseases
UN	United Nations
UNAIDS	Joint United Nations Programme on HIV/AIDS
UNICEF	United Nations Children's Fund

USAID	United States Agency for International Development
VBCRC	Vector Biology and Control Research Centre
WHO	World Health Organization
WHO AFRO	World Health Organization Regional Office for Africa
WHOPES	World Health Organization Pesticide Evaluation Scheme

Nothing But Nets

Introduction

Making Evidence-Based Global Health in Africa

Birds chirp over a black background. What Spotify might call "African tribal music" begins to swell. "Mosquitoes kill **millions** of people every year," the text reads, as a sunlit African savannah materializes on screen. Transported to a dusty village road where a child clutches chickens in both hands, we read that mosquitoes spread malaria across the continent, devastating families and communities. "We lose a child to the disease every 30 seconds." Cut to a water collection site, a bright-eyed young girl is in the foreground. "But not **her**. She sleeps under a **bed net**." A blue meshwork enshrouds a woman and her baby. They peek out from underneath. "It stops mosquitoes. Protecting her and those she loves." Text and images roll past in a steady rhythm. "Bed Nets Save Lives." "Send a **Net**. Save a **Life**." More calls to action follow: "provide hope," "save a family," "save a village," "buy a bed net." Country by country a map of Africa is pieced together, an isolated orange mass in a sea of black: "Together we can cover a continent . . ." Finally, the music recedes, leaving us with a calling card: NothingButNets.net.[1]

Since Nothing But Nets made its 2006 YouTube debut, the charity (now called United to Beat Malaria) has procured over 13 million insecticide-treated bed nets for people living in malaria-endemic areas, primarily in sub-Saharan Africa.[2] It has not acted alone. Since 2000 an array of nongovernmental organizations (NGOs), philanthropies, private companies, multilateral agencies, and wealthy countries have helped deliver over one billion insecticide-treated nets (ITNs) on the continent. Like them, Nothing But Nets has justified its intense focus on nets by citing the health intervention's ability to save lives. The charity has additionally sold supporters on donating nets by invoking the technology's simplicity and low cost. For $10 you can "send a net" to "save a life." "Talk about a net profit," as the charity's founder, the sports columnist Rick Reilly, would say.[3]

The video, the slogans, and the puns present this object as an easy and self-evident means of preventing a deadly disease. Very simply, these mesh bed coverings provide a physical and chemical barrier that can block, repel, and kill malaria-carrying *Anopheles* mosquitoes, many species of which bite at night. The nets protect individuals sleeping underneath them and, if used in enough households, can help reduce malaria transmission in a given region. This image, however, belies the fact that ITNs—what they are, how they work, and how they became something organizations wanted to "cover" the African continent with—are anything but straightforward. The process by which the world came to understand them as universally applicable life-saving tools and a preferred method for controlling malaria in the twenty-first century is the subject of this book.

When health officials first considered using ITNs for malaria control in the early 1980s, few would have predicted that these objects would become a major global health intervention. Despite the tool's seemingly obvious public health utility, entomologists were unsure whether rips in a net would still allow mosquitoes to reach sleepers, rendering the insecticide futile. Furthermore, they had outstanding questions about the relationship between malaria infection and disease. If nets spared young children some but not all infective mosquito bites, would those children still suffer severe symptoms or death? Malaria-endemic areas also varied considerably, prompting questions about whether ITNs could achieve the same effects in different social, ecological, and epidemiological settings. Even in 1991, when scientists published experimental data showing that the technology helped reduce child mortality, representatives of the World Health Organization (WHO) questioned whether these results applied everywhere. ITNs remained marginal among malaria control strategies until 1998, when the WHO and a cadre of development agencies made the technology a centerpiece of a new partnership called Roll Back Malaria. How did this transformation occur? And what does the ascendance of ITNs tell us about the development of our contemporary global health enterprise over the past forty years?

Public health specialists and scholars have offered some preliminary answers to these questions. Malaria experts have cited the effectiveness of the scientific process, specifically randomized controlled trials, in proving that

ITNs could save lives the same way everywhere. These experts claimed that the application of "evidence based" practices—of which randomized controlled trials are the gold standard—objectively demonstrated the technology's biomedical utility, making it an obvious candidate for global health funding.[4] Historians of malaria control, on the other hand, have explained the widespread adoption of ITNs by invoking the influence of neoliberal ideology and an emphasis on "magic-bullet" solutions in malaria control and global health more generally.[5] Leaders of major health and development agencies embraced the intervention because it put responsibility for public health into the hands of individual consumers, who could reduce malaria by buying and using ITNs themselves. This in turn made it unnecessary for these agencies to deal with conditions of systemic poverty, which perpetuate malaria. In the first account, ITNs appear to be a resounding success and model for the development of other evidence-based public health interventions. In the second account, ITNs are just one more imperfect solution to deep structural problems resulting from long-standing political and economic inequalities.

Both accounts are useful in understanding how this intervention became a centerpiece of global malaria control; however, neither is entirely sufficient. That is because neither recognizes ITNs as dynamic historical objects that people defined and used differently over time. Entomologists initially dominated investigations of this technology, measuring the effects of nets on mosquitoes rather than on human disease. Only in the mid-1980s, after scientists with backgrounds in clinical research and epidemiology began to measure the technology's effects on human disease—an incredibly complicated and contingent task—did they begin to define ITNs as medical objects suitable for testing in randomized controlled trials. Research teams had to conduct many of these biomedical experiments across Africa to demonstrate that ITNs reduced child mortality everywhere, since the mechanism by which nets saved lives remained obscure. Even in the early 1990s, before research teams completed those randomized controlled mortality trials, African health officials, research teams, and NGOs started disseminating the tool on a small scale. The intervention seemed to them to be a financially and practically feasible way for African countries to mitigate malaria in an era of diminished resources. In other words, factors other than biomedical efficacy and global policies compelled groups to adopt ITNs in Africa long before major health and development agencies championed the intervention.

By historicizing the rise of one of the most celebrated global health interventions of the twenty-first century, this book provides a new lens on the history of global health—one that attends to people's use and understanding of material things. Thus far, scholars have focused on the activities and policies of influential institutions to explain the popularity of individualized technological solutions in global health. In doing so, they have often framed these technological solutions as proxies for groups' broader political-economic interests rather than materials with distinct trajectories, affordances, and effects. Many studies show how pharmaceuticals, vaccines, and ready-to-use therapeutic food target disease in a narrowly technical and biomedical fashion without addressing the underlying social and economic determinants of health.[6] Fewer studies consider the ways that shifting historical circumstances have shaped understandings of these technologies, their physical attributes, and their application over time.[7] By paying greater attention to this material dimension, this book illustrates that global health technologies are not interchangeable means of accomplishing the same political ends. Rather, these technologies have specific and evolving characteristics, which affect how and why people deploy them for large-scale public health.

The history of ITNs also enhances understandings of the development of global malaria control, an endeavor in which nets now play a starring role. Scientists began investigating the technology for large-scale malaria control just over a decade after the WHO ended its Malaria Eradication Programme in 1969. Among other things, this eradication program precipitated the spread of resistance to pesticides and drugs and provided fodder for criticism of top-down, disease-specific campaigns. Political and financial support for malaria control—now seen as an expensive and uncertain investment—declined sharply. This lack of resources proved disastrous as malaria rates rebounded in places that had to stop eradication activities prematurely and as resistance to the cheap antimalarial drug chloroquine began to spread worldwide. During the 1980s, moreover, governments of many malaria-affected countries struggled to follow the sometimes-competing directives of international agencies, which pressured them to cut health sector spending under structural adjustment policies and to build up primary health care services. Malaria control activities were subsumed under inadequately resourced primary health care projects or under the private sector in many places. The growing malaria crisis was exacerbated by the HIV/AIDS pandemic, which drew significantly greater attention and funding. As the task of malaria control took on new political, economic, and epidemiological dimensions during the 1980s and 1990s, scientists, health officials, and donor agencies collectively reimagined how ITNs would mitigate the problems facing malaria-endemic countries. The fact that this technology became enshrined as a lifesaving, evidence-based intervention and a cornerstone of global malaria control was not inevitable. This development proved incredibly influential, however, drawing into malaria activities a host of new organizations, not all of which were familiar with the complexities of this disease.

Finally, by historicizing ITNs, this book sheds light on the key roles that African populations have played in the development of evidence-based global health. As home to roughly 90% of the world's malaria burden, sub-Saharan Africa became the main target for global malaria control activities, including ITN research and implementation. The epidemiology and ecology of malaria as well as the public health and research infrastructure in African research sites informed how and why scientists carried out bed net experiments there. Teams of African and expatriate scientists adjusted their research questions, experimental protocols, and scientific practices to trial participants' use of bed nets, relying on local health workers and other intermediaries from study areas to do so.[8] These experiments generated generalizable biomedical knowledge that nets saved lives, which policy makers used to attract international investment in malaria control and authorize ITN distribution around the world. Yet when African health officials and their partners adopted global recommendations, they had to modify domestic distribution efforts as citizens took up the intervention in uneven and unanticipated ways, all while navigating the offers and demands of external donors. Turning ITNs into an evidence-based global health intervention was a highly contingent and African affair, one in which locally situated knowledge and practices were continually translated into global health knowledge and strategies, and vice versa.

Objects of Global Health: A Biographical Approach

This book traces the development of insecticide-treated nets into a major global health intervention by following the object's biography as it unfolded on a transnational scale and in Kenya—a key site of ITN activities—since 1980. A biographical approach emphasizes that objects do not have an inherent, stable, or singular identity, as if they exist independently of history or society.[9] Rather, people imbue objects with different functions, significance, and meanings as they use and structure their activities around these objects in different contexts. Before research teams demonstrated that ITNs could reduce child mortality, for example, the international community paid little attention to these objects, and ordinary (untreated) bed nets continued to circulate as luxury goods in many African countries. After scientists reconceptualized ITNs as lifesaving tools through randomized controlled trials, however, patrons and policy makers promoted the same technology as a solution for both disease prevention and economic development in Africa. Nets' new identity opened the floodgates for investment in malaria control after decades of international inaction, transforming what had been a luxury good into a common charity item and fixture in many poor, rural households on the continent.[10] ITNs acquired different identities at different moments and in different contexts, based as much on the practices of African populations as on those of donors, policy makers, and researchers from the global north. Although understandings of this technology and its function were highly malleable—more so, for example, compared to vaccines—certain of these understandings prevailed and significantly shaped the technology's global trajectory. This book explores how those conceptions, or identities, crystallized and what they potentiated or foreclosed in efforts to control malaria in Africa.

The biography of ITNs was heavily influenced by changes in international health and development over the late twentieth century. After World War II the WHO and other United Nations (UN) agencies held significant influence in authorizing and directing public health campaigns based on the votes and donations of member states. At the end of the 1970s, the WHO sought to respond to the needs of newly decolonized countries by prioritizing basic health care for all and integrating health and socioeconomic concerns. The global debt crisis of the 1980s, however, seriously weakened this system of international health governance and financing as well as burgeoning calls for international health equity. The World Bank and International Monetary Fund began floating structural adjustment loans to indebted countries— many of them former colonies—requiring the countries to adopt a variety of austerity measures and trade liberalization policies. The World Bank and some wealthy countries, most notably the United States, vocally criticized the ability of state-based bureaucracies to use resources efficiently and effectively. As a result, these donors channeled more and more of their foreign aid through nongovernmental and private organizations, rather than directly to recipient governments or the WHO. By the early 1990s, the World Bank had become the largest funder of international health activities, doling out resources based on principles of cost efficiency, accountability, and market fundamentalism as well as economic valuations of life and health. International health leaders continued to focus on the health of the world's poor, but they increasingly addressed these concerns through neoliberal policies that leveraged market mechanisms and nongovernmental channels to deliver health care in a decentralized fashion.[11]

This period of retraction and restructuring gave way to a renaissance in what became known as "global health" at the turn of the twenty-first century.[12] Public-private partnerships became a popular form of cost sharing for public health efforts. The Roll Back Malaria partnership, launched by the WHO, World Bank, United Nations Children's Fund, and United Nations Development Programme, served as a prominent example. Funding for global health skyrocketed as new donors, such as the Bill and Melinda Gates Foundation, became involved. Humanitarian organizations entered the field in droves to fill in resource and governance gaps in low-income regions. No longer able to justify investments in foreign aid under the banner of fighting communism, the United States levied substantial funds during the post–Cold War period in the name of global health security. The United States and other donors also found ways to bypass the state-based UN system and track their investments with more accountability through private voluntary organizations, multinational commodity funds, and other such mechanisms. Meanwhile, leaders of major health and development agencies made the case that protecting health stimulated economic development. Saving lives by reducing disease and disability meant more workers and more consumers. Advocates made this case incredibly successfully for malaria, one of the only diseases mentioned specifically (alongside HIV/AIDS) in the UN Millennium Development Goals, introduced in 2000.

Epistemological changes also had consequences for this new regime of global health. Statistical, experimental, and epidemiological models of evidence, which characterize "evidence-based" clinical practice, became the predominant means of evaluating public health interventions.[13] Scientists and practitioners embraced randomized controlled trials to deal with nonstandard variation among research subjects and settings and to provide probabilistic certainty that an intervention would be medically efficacious elsewhere, even in cases where the mechanism of action—or the scientific reason that a medical intervention worked—remained uncertain. For example, scientists did not know exactly how ITNs reduced child mortality when they carried out randomized controlled trials with the intervention. Moreover, this knowledge seemed unnecessary to them once statistics showed that the technology saved lives. Just as efforts to cut health care costs facilitated the use of evidence-based practices in the hospitals and health systems of industrialized countries, donors and policy makers privileged interventions that were substantiated by randomized controlled trials to rationalize global health investments. The experimental paradigm provided confidence that an intervention would pay off in years of healthy life and, for manufacturers and distributors, in profits as well.

The life of ITNs was interwoven with these broad shifts, as the technology transformed from a cheap stopgap measure for malaria, to a universally applicable evidence-based intervention, to a seemingly wise investment of health and development resources. The object thus serves as a kind of "traceable dye" through the complex circuitry of global health as it operated within and between distant locales, from Kenyan villages to conference rooms in Abuja, Geneva, and Washington, DC.[14] While the specific nature of malaria and ITNs affected the way that people defined this object over time, people imagined and interacted with it in a larger world of health goods. This world also included the infrastructure that health authorities used to test and distribute these goods: networks of village health workers, maternal and child health clinics, epidemiological data, and global commodity funds. People's experiences with oral rehydration tablets, birth control pills, antiretroviral therapy, vaccines, vitamin A supplementation, condoms, and other tools directly informed their interactions with ITNs. Conversely, people's experiences with ITNs inspired efforts to make, promote, and disseminate other health interventions. ITNs inhabited a dense world filled with material things as well as nonmaterial social, political, and economic relations. The biography of this technology, then, is not merely a story of a single tool or efforts to control a single disease; it is a story about the development of evidence-based global health as refracted through various objects and infrastructures that came to animate this enterprise.

Viewing ITNs as part of this larger tapestry sheds new light on the way evidence-based global health operates not only as a scientific activity but also as a capitalist one. As with other evidence-based interventions, randomized controlled trial results and cost-effectiveness calculations abstracted ITNs from the contexts in which African populations used them, thus making them "generic objects" deemed to work regardless of local circumstances or needs.[15] These statistical findings also standardized a use value for nets as devices that saved lives anywhere at a very low cost—a utility desired by major donor agencies.[16] This in turn rendered nets commutable in a larger economy of lifesaving global health goods, a marketplace in which the intervention appeared competitive with things like childhood vaccines. A variety of organizations—from narrowly focused charities such as Nothing But Nets to the US government and World Bank—began procuring and circulating ITNs en masse through international markets and local distribution channels across Africa based on this utility. In this way, the scientific practices at the heart of evidence-based global health transformed ITNs into global health commodities, which have further integrated disparate non-Western localities into worldwide networks of capitalist exchange.[17]

This transformation had multiple effects on efforts to control malaria. For one thing, it obscured many of the lessons scientists learned when they conducted trials during the 1980s and 1990s: local contingencies of ITN use could affect whether and to what extent the technology reduced mortality. Overlooking such concerns helped accelerate the dissemination of ITNs across Africa and the global south as donors sent nets to save lives and, in the process, to promote economic development. The popularity of pay-for-performance funding mechanisms, where countries are rewarded with additional resources for distributing nets and other health goods, reinforced the circulation of ITNs as global health commodities. Moreover, the massive increase in demand for ITNs stimulated manufacturing, particularly among multinational textile and chemical companies capable of making products that met regulatory standards. Most African textile companies as well as local tailors in rural areas have not benefited much from this new demand, because they are unable to make ITNs at scale, to meet regulatory standards, or to compete for global tenders.[18] More fundamentally, the machinery of evidence-based global health that transformed ITNs into global health commodities has perpetuated paradigms of fighting malaria at the level of individual consumers. As experiences from Africa show, such paradigms can be quite precarious in a climate of volatile, unpredictable global health aid.[19]

Methods and Structure of the Book

Like people, objects lead multifaceted lives that can be difficult to capture in a single, coherent biography.[20] I have chosen to concentrate on aspects of insecticide-treated nets' life history that help explain the intervention's rise to prominence and the consequences of that development but also address broader questions about how global health interventions are constructed, adopted into health policy, and implemented in practice. I am especially interested in the interplay between the ways people conceptualize, use, and govern public health interventions, a dynamic often overlooked in histories of global health institutions and programs. Greater attention to this interplay can enhance understandings of why policy makers and health officials choose certain interventions and distribute them in certain ways. I use approaches and methods from the history and sociology of science and technology to provide this attention.

Furthermore, I examine the biography of ITNs largely as it played out in or in relation to Africa insofar as the continent has been the main site for bed net research and distribution. I describe activities in multiple African countries that influenced developments with the intervention and with global malaria control. Moving across these sites helps illuminate some of the ways in which knowledge and practices circulate (or not) in global health programs. I also focus specifically on Kenya, a prominent site of ITN research and implementation. In some ways Kenya's experience was exemplary of what happened with ITNs across the continent; in other ways it was singularly influential. As in many African countries, for instance, Kenyan health officials initially tried to scale up nets through social marketing programs on the recommendation of Roll Back Malaria partners. Around 2007, Kenyan scientists and their expatriate partners published research showing that people used the intervention in greater numbers and with a greater public health impact if they were given the nets for free; the WHO cited this research in recommending free mass distribution campaigns as the new ideal. Periodically zooming in on Kenya's experience provides a more detailed look into the relationship between specific social, cultural, political, and economic circumstances and the development of global health knowledge and technologies. Kenyan history, and not just the history of wealthy institutions from the global north, helps us understand the history of ITNs and evidence-based global health.

Defining ITNs as an evidence-based malaria control intervention was a collective and transnational effort involving a diverse range of people, from residents of rural villages to leaders of multinational agencies. These people operated in various settings and at various scales of governance. It is impossible to capture the perspectives of everyone or even most of those involved in this history. I draw on a combination of archival and published material, oral histories, and participant observation from three continents to trace the broad historical arc of ITNs while still grounding this history in people's specific experiences. I consulted the archives of the WHO, World Bank, US Agency for International Development, UN, London School of Hygiene and Tropical Medicine, Centers for Disease Control and Prevention (CDC) in the United States, and the Kenya Medical Research Institute (KEMRI)-Centre for Global Health Research to gain insight into the priorities, decisions, and bureaucratic practices of many of the institutions involved in bed net activities. I complemented my reading of official documents by interviewing scientists, health officials, malaria control advocates, and community health workers from Kenya, North America, and Europe. This allowed me to get a more detailed perspective on how bed net research, policy making, and implementation operated on the ground, as well as to understand what my interviewees felt was most important about this intervention and its history. During my time in Kenya in 2015–2016, I interviewed residents of Siaya, Kisii, and Kisumu Counties with the help of my research assistant, Molly Omany, to gain insight into how Kenyans understood and experienced ITN research and distribution. I chose these counties because they were important sites for research on the efficacy and distribution of ITNs. While in Kenya, I was also able to see how people used bed nets, how the government and their nongovernmental partners advertised the intervention, and how local health workers distributed nets through routine channels (like clinics) and a coordinated distribution campaign. I recognize that these sources do not provide a complete historical picture and that my collection of sources was contingent on many factors, including my interviewees' perceptions of me and my project, and their own interests and constraints in sharing their experiences. Nonetheless, by reading and weaving these sources together, I hope to provide a window into the multidirectional influences on and consequences of global health objects.

This book follows ITNs (in their various iterations) through three important domains of the object's life as an evidence-based global health intervention:

research, policy making, and implementation.[21] While certain of these activities preceded others, there was also significant overlap and interaction between them. Health officials, for example, did not always wait for scientific consensus or official global policy to implement ITNs in African villages. The chapters artificially separate these domains for analytic clarity, occasionally doubling back to examine another facet of ITNs' evolving identity. In building up these layers, the book stresses that science, policy, and implementation inform each other in evidence-based global health, but not necessarily in the neat linear progression that advocates portray.

The first two chapters examine the history of ITN research in Africa during the 1980s and 1990s to see how and why this object became understood as a universally applicable lifesaving tool. Chapter 1 begins the biography by examining the emergence of ITNs as objects of scientific inquiry, or "scientific objects," during the 1980s.[22] It illustrates how the politics of late twentieth-century global health and development, along with local populations and conditions in African research sites, shaped the production of scientific knowledge about this intervention. Seeking a cost-effective solution to a growing public health crisis, scientists studied the ability of ITNs to reduce malaria transmission, disease, and child mortality in impoverished, rural areas. This research inspired a series of randomized controlled trials across Africa, trials that reconceptualized ITNs as tools that protected individual users in the same way regardless of local ecologies, health systems, or sociocultural circumstances.

Chapter 2 delves into the last and largest bed net efficacy trial ever conducted to see how ITNs finally became consolidated as universally applicable biomedical technologies seen as capable of saving children's lives in any setting. Conducted by the CDC and KEMRI in Siaya, Kenya, during the late 1990s, this trial addressed outstanding concerns about the viability of the intervention in areas of intense, year-round malaria transmission. Local conditions, practices, and beliefs in Siaya significantly shaped the production of biomedical knowledge about ITNs. The contingency of these local circumstances on the object's effectiveness as a lifesaving tool got lost, however, as scientists generalized findings into global health knowledge.

As ITNs gained notoriety in scientific circles, the intervention became a common fixture in malaria control policy discussions during the 1990s. Chapter 3 explores how and why international and Kenyan health officials incorporated the intervention into global and national malaria control policies, respectively. Global health leaders lauded ITNs as "evidence-based" interventions when they adopted them in Roll Back Malaria, a new program created at the close of the twentieth century. Such suggestions that scientific evidence catalyzed the tool's uptake, however, overlook the fact that earlier calls to adopt the technology in Kenya and other African countries sometimes preceded the circulation of scientific knowledge. The tool's suitability for decentralized and privatized health systems—not just evidence of its biomedical efficacy—informed policy makers' decision to include ITNs in malaria control policy.

In 1998 the WHO officially launched Roll Back Malaria in Africa, the organization's first malaria-specific program since its malaria eradication campaign of the 1950s and 1960s. Chapters 4 and 5 track the life of ITNs as health officials and their partners deployed the intervention in Africa under the banner of Roll Back Malaria. Chapter 4 tracks health officials' implementation of ITN policies in Africa during the 2000s. Since major donors to Roll Back Malaria prioritized economic efficiency, accountability, and sustainability, the program's leaders adopted market-based strategies to distribute nets. Such strategies rested on a conception of ITNs as universally applicable lifesaving tools. These strategies also operated under the false assumption that poor, at-risk populations would inherently understand and prioritize the lifesaving value of this technology and they ignored the diversity in local ecologies of malaria in Africa. Tracking the challenges that African health officials faced in implementing globally sanctioned bed net strategies in Tanzania and Zambia—two places that policy makers held up as models for bed net distribution at different points over the decade—this chapter reveals how the identity of ITNs as global health commodities led to ineffective and precarious malaria control efforts during the first decade of Roll Back Malaria.

Chapter 5 examines ITNs as a domestic technology that Kenyan populations have adopted in their daily lives as bed net distribution has expanded over the twenty-first century. Kenyan health officials and scientists discovered that, for various economic, social, and epistemological reasons, few people at risk for malaria were buying or using ITNs. Showing statistically that more people in Kenya used nets when these were given to them for free, these scientists produced knowledge to justify free mass bed net distribution

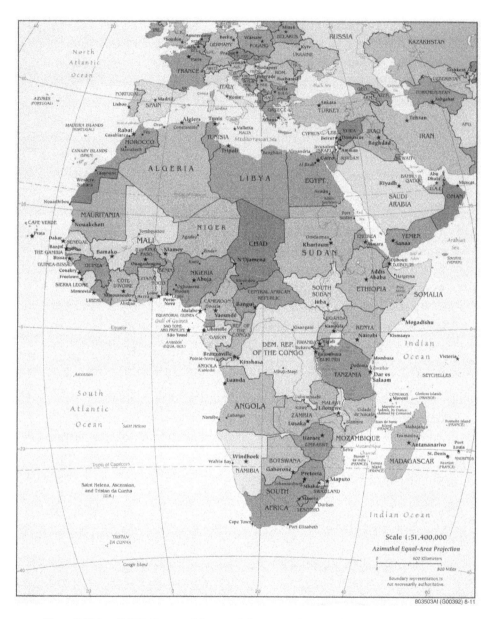

Map of Africa (2011). Source: Library of Congress Geography and Map Division

campaigns across the continent. Resolving the issue of cost, however, did not solve all the problems involved in using an individualized tool to combat malaria.

I conclude by looking at the current status and challenges of malaria control in Africa, which continues to rely heavily on ITNs. I will also discuss some of the implications of the rise of ITNs as a main method of malaria control on the continent, including the technology's effects on the environment, mosquito populations, malaria rates, and public health systems. Finally, I offer a short summation of the lessons for contemporary global health practice provided by the history of ITNs and the history of global health technologies more generally. These lessons will be important to keep in mind as insecticide resistance increases across the continent and new tools, such as malaria vaccines, become incorporated into the malaria control arsenal.

1

The Scientific Object

Becoming the Right Tool for the Job

On the surface, the history of insecticide-treated nets reads like a rags-to-riches tale in evidence-based public health, in which rigorous epidemiological experiments transformed a mundane, low-tech tool into a prominent global health intervention. In the 1970s, before scientists subjected ITNs to experimental scrutiny, few public health officials paid much attention to bed nets, which did not seem to be obvious candidates for large-scale malaria control. Following a series of successful randomized controlled trials in Africa during the 1990s, policy makers began citing statistical findings that nets reduced child mortality, in order to justify the intervention's wide distribution. In this cursory account, science, and epidemiology in particular, appears to be a chief catalyst and driving force.

A closer examination of ITNs' life as "scientific objects"—objects systematically observed and tested for their impact on mosquitoes and malaria—reveals a much more complicated and contingent story.[1] Scientists first became interested in the intervention at the beginning of the 1980s, against a backdrop of dwindling financial support and technical resources for malaria control. Until then, populations around the world had used ordinary (untreated) bed nets for a variety of purposes, including but not limited to disease prevention. Scientists' interest was not spurred by confidence that nets were the best way to preserve people's health, especially in rural sub-Saharan Africa, where malaria transmission tended to be especially intense and adequate public health infrastructure was lacking. Rather, conditions of resource scarcity, compounded by a global economic crisis and externally applied austerity measures in low-income countries, largely informed how and why scientists studied this cheap, seemingly simple tool. They investigated the feasibility of incorporating ITNs into impoverished African health systems and inchoate primary health care programs as much as the efficacy of nets themselves. Defining ITNs as scientific objects was not merely a technical exercise of knowledge production; it was an endeavor deeply entangled with the politics and practicalities of international health and development in Africa.

This context, along with environmental and sociocultural conditions in research sites, in turn shaped ITN experiments and their results. National health systems, the built infrastructure in study areas, and mosquito ecologies all influenced scientists' activities and findings. African populations, including study participants, village leaders, and village health workers, also came to ITN research with their own sociocultural practices and understandings of bed nets. Their interactions with both nets and research teams influenced who used ITNs and how they did so, informing study results as well. Evidence—the most influential of which was produced in Africa—for the efficacy of ITNs was incredibly contingent on local circumstances.

Throughout the 1980s, scientists recognized these contingencies in their studies, often qualifying their results as applicable only to certain national or epidemiological situations. This dovetailed with prevailing notions among malaria experts that malaria was a focal disease, which was transmitted differently in different areas due to a variety of ecological and social factors. The applied orientation of many experiments also led scientists to qualify claims of generalizability. This was true for the first trial measuring ITNs' ability to reduce child mortality, launched in The Gambia in 1988; the trial was framed as informing public health activities in that country and not malaria-endemic areas more broadly.

This focus on local contingencies and specificity soon began to shift. In the early 1990s, promising findings from The Gambia combined with renewed urgency around malaria control in Africa prompted research teams to conduct four large-scale randomized controlled trials on the continent. They aimed to show that ITNs could save lives regardless of local ecologies, health systems, or sociocultural circumstances. In the process, these randomized controlled trials helped reconstitute malaria chiefly as a biomedical problem amenable to such an individualized and standardized technological solution. Over the decade, ITNs and the task of controlling malaria came to mutually define each other, and these inexpensive, politically salient devices transformed into "the right tool for the job."[2] An explication of the trajectory of ITNs as scientific objects reveals how this change occurred as practices from evidence-based medicine became increasingly incorporated into public health.[3]

Coming of Age after Malaria Eradication

Changes in international health and malaria control during the 1960s and 1970s shaped scientists' interest in using insecticide-treated nets on a population-wide scale in Africa. Dwindling technical and financial resources for malaria programming played an influential role. The World Health Organization (WHO) had officially abandoned its Malaria Eradication Programme in 1969 as both the organization and participating governments ran low on funds to support the struggling campaign. Over the course of the program, moreover, *Anopheles* mosquitoes in many parts of the world became resistant to the pesticide dichlorodiphenyltrichloroethane (DDT). Indoor residual insecticide spraying, which had been the centerpiece of eradication activities, fell out of favor as a result. Even though the WHO did not extend eradication activities to most of sub-Saharan Africa, smaller tests with indoor residual spraying on the continent suggested that this expensive, intensive method would not work as a long-term solution to malaria anyway.[4] The Garki Project, conducted in northern Nigeria from 1969–1976, was particularly discouraging; it showed that even a perfectly designed DDT spraying program combined with mass drug administration could not interrupt malaria transmission.[5] Giving up on global malaria eradication, leaders of the international health community embraced malaria control as a new goal. At the same time, they rejected top-down, one-size-fits-all approaches epitomized by DDT spraying campaigns.

Backlash against these approaches coincided with broader shifts in international health and development, including increased interest in rural development and the primary health care movement. Advocates of primary health care, such as the WHO director-general, Halfdan Mahler, promoted decentralized health care targeted toward meeting people's basic needs, rather than vertical disease control campaigns or expensive tertiary care. In line with this ethos, the WHO recommended that African governments integrate malaria control into basic health services, especially in rural areas where malaria burdens were highest.[6] Primary health care advocates emphasized the compatibility of antimalarial drug treatment and chemoprophylaxis with the integrated model, which privileged the dispensation of drugs to combat multiple disease threats in low-income settings. Integrated malaria control programs thus privileged pharmaceuticals for malaria control in Africa.[7]

The changing tides of the global economy also shaped the way that international health officials and African governments pursued malaria control in the post-eradication period. The oil shocks and high levels of inflation of the 1970s helped generate a major global recession. The recession hurt the economies of major manufacturing countries in the global north as well as in commodity-exporting, low-income countries that had accumulated high levels of debt. The World Bank and International Monetary Fund (IMF) provided structural adjustment loans to the latter group—including many African countries—in danger of defaulting on their debt. In return, these recipients had to restructure their economies by implementing a variety of austerity measures and trade liberalization policies. Consequently, many African governments cut health care spending and began privatizing health services. With some exceptions, at-risk populations relied heavily on private sector channels to access antimalarial drugs and other malaria control tools.[8]

Health and development organizations adjusted their aid priorities and strategies in this era of diminishing resources. Although Mahler and the WHO pushed for broad-based primary health care, members of other donor agencies, including the Rockefeller Foundation, World Bank, and United Nations Children's Fund (UNICEF) thought such a project was unrealistically expensive. As an alternative, they called for selective approaches to primary health care justified through metrics measuring the cost per death averted, or "cost-effectiveness." Selective primary health care, as the approach was called, privileged simple, inexpensive, individualized technologies that could be distributed in decentralized health systems, such as oral rehydration therapy, "essential medicines," and vaccines for childhood diseases.[9] These types of technologies, which many donors dubbed and embraced as "appropriate technologies" during this period, were supposed to extend health care into poor, rural areas using limited resources.[10] This further reinforced African health programs' heavy reliance on the cheap antimalarial drug chloroquine, among other health commodities.

At the same time, malaria experts and health officials' conceptions of malaria changed in the wake of global malaria eradication, due in large part to experiences and challenges with DDT spraying campaigns. They adopted the view that malaria was a focal disease whose characteristics depended on local social, economic, and ecological factors, since these affected the ways in which people came in contact with mosquitoes.[11] Experts incorporated this view into a new "epidemiological approach" to malaria, which "recogniz[ed] the variability of epidemiological risks at local level" and stratified areas by epidemiological characteristics, such as the seasonality and stability of malaria transmission.[12] In this approach, one had to consider (and theoretically control) malaria differently in regions with endemic, year-round malaria transmission than in regions where malaria emerged in sporadic epidemics or only during the rainy season. Local variability mattered.

In 1979 WHO officials incorporated this newfound attention to variability into a strategy called "Tactical Variants."[13] This strategy established four sets of recommendations for malaria control for different epidemiological strata. Officials placed most countries in sub-Saharan Africa into Tactical Variant I, the stratum farthest from malaria eradication. They recommended that these countries focus solely on reducing mortality through drug treatment—or, as one official dubbed it, "palliative measures."[14] Like calls for integrated malaria control in primary health care programs, the Tactical Variants framework encouraged WHO member states in Africa to adopt pharmaceutical-based malaria control strategies to hold the line against the deadly disease.

Around the same time that WHO officials recommended that African countries embrace drug treatment as the basis of their malaria control programs, however, chloroquine resistance began to emerge on the continent. This development was especially disheartening because African countries and rural communities had benefited substantially from the drug throughout the 1960s and 1970s. Chloroquine-resistant strains of *Plasmodium falciparum*—the deadliest malaria parasite species and most common species in Africa—first appeared in Southeast Asia in 1957; resistant strains later appeared in East Africa around 1978. Chloroquine resistance initially proliferated in places where health officials included mass drug administration in eradication activities. The overprescription of chloroquine for fever or as a prophylactic exacerbated the spread of resistance, as did people not receiving or taking a full course of the drug.[15] Some countries adopted second- and third-line drugs, such as sulfadoxine-pyrimethamine, which were more expensive. Health programmers who previously relied on mass chemoprophylaxis began limiting the practice to certain vulnerable groups, such as pregnant women or young children, to slow the spread of chloroquine resistance.[16]

In practice, due to a lack of resources, international and African national health officials were constrained in their attempts to reduce reliance on the cheap drug. Donors who previously contributed great sums of money to malaria eradication grew skeptical about the viability of malaria control activities and pulled their funding from the cause as a result.[17] The recession undoubtedly discouraged investment in malaria control as well, since the problem did not directly affect wealthy, industrialized countries of the global north. Beginning in the 1960s, advances in immunology and molecular biology sparked interest around malaria vaccines. Developing a malaria vaccine was not as easy as scientists had hoped, however, and they realized they would have to pursue other options in the meantime.

Due partly to this technological and economic retraction, malaria began to resurge around the world. Populations that had benefited from eradication activities and reduced malaria transmission lost their immunity to the disease. Consequently, in places where insecticide-spraying teams stopped eradication activities prematurely, people suffered from epidemics of severe, fatal forms of malaria. This "rebound effect" threatened populations in many regions across the global south. Although chloroquine continued to be effective in most parts of Africa during the first half of the 1980s, African health officials faced the prospect of a similar deadly upsurge. The withdrawal of funding for malaria, which encouraged dependence on chloroquine, likely accelerated this development. The escalating HIV/AIDS pandemic, economic downturn, and divestment of national health systems exacerbated malaria mortality across the continent as well. International and African health officials faced an impending malaria crisis on the continent just as they lost most of the tools and resources to mitigate it.

Becoming a Scientific Object: Early Investigations of ITNs

Against this backdrop, scientists and health officials started to identify insecticide-treated nets as a potential stopgap measure. Despite garnering new attention in this period, however, bed nets were not entirely novel technologies. People had slept under nets for centuries. In the fifth century BCE the Greek historian Herodotus described how Egyptians slept under fishing nets to protect themselves from swarms of gnats. Populations around the world—including communities in China, Japan, West Africa, India, Paraguay, and Papua New Guinea—also slept under nets and other coverings, sometimes but not always for protection from insect pests.[18] Nineteenth-century

European colonizers not only noted such practices in their writings but also used nets to protect themselves from pesky mosquitoes while stationed in warm climates. Some even claimed that nets protected sleepers from noxious marsh miasmas, understood at the time as the cause of malaria.[19] After Sir Ronald Ross elaborated the link between mosquitoes and malaria at the beginning of the twentieth century, people increasingly slept under bed nets specifically to prevent malaria. By mid-century, some had even combined ordinary bed nets with insecticide to ward off mosquitoes. The United States and Russian militaries, for example, used DDT-treated bed nets during World War II, as did residents of China's Yunnan Province as early as the 1950s.[20]

ITNs of the 1980s, however, were distinct from their predecessors in one important way: they included newly developed pyrethroid insecticides. Following the backlash against DDT, including the US ban of the pesticide in 1972, chemists focused on finding alternatives. Michael Elliot and colleagues at the Rothamsted Experimental Station in England focused on this new class of insecticides called pyrethroids, synthetic analogues to the natural insecticide pyrethrum. In 1972 they developed permethrin, a pyrethroid that was effective against many insects, had low mammalian and avian toxicity, and did not degrade in air and light as quickly as other pyrethroids.[21] Although permethrin could not compete commercially with other insecticides on the market, which were used largely in agriculture, both it and deltamethrin (discovered in 1974) provided new opportunities for public health. This included, as one scientist put it, a "revived interest in bednets."[22]

On a 1982 visit to China a malaria specialist with the WHO, Lee Self, raised the idea of treating bed nets with pyrethroids. This idea was partly inspired by American soldiers' use of permethrin-coated clothing while stationed in tropical regions.[23] Members of the WHO Expert Committee on Vector Biology and Control deemed this strategy worthy of consideration, seeking methods that non-health professionals could carry out with little financial and technical support to "improve the long-term effectiveness of the control of vectorborne diseases and to achieve economies" in endemic areas.[24] For these malaria experts, it seemed intuitive that ITNs could prevent malaria by blocking, repelling, and even killing mosquitoes.

Shortly after Self's 1982 visit, East Asia and the Western Pacific, where Self worked, became a locus of ITN activities. China in particular adopted pyrethroid-treated nets in public health programs early on, partly because of residents' familiarity with the technology. Not only had residents of Yunnan Province used DDT-treated bed nets decades earlier, but residents of other malaria-endemic provinces had also been using ordinary bed nets (among other methods) to prevent malaria for many years. "Barefoot doctors" helped carry out these activities at the commune level as part of China's primary health care system.[25] In these regions local tailors manufactured bed nets, which individuals then purchased to protect themselves from mosquitoes. Chinese scientists introduced pyrethroid-treated nets into this existing infrastructure, looking for an alternative vector control measure to indoor residual spraying.[26]

ITNs fit well into China's robust, community-level public health system. Residents would bring their own bed nets to a specific meeting place where local health workers concocted a solution of water and deltamethrin emulsifiable concentrate. Using their own wash bins, people would soak their nets in the insecticide solution and hang the nets to dry.[27] This process depended heavily on both residents and local health workers, who calculated the amount of water and insecticide required to coat the nets. While people purchased their bed nets, the Chinese government provided the insecticide for free.[28] This system worked well in China, providing a model for ITN programs elsewhere, which similarly called on residents to pay for at least part of this public health intervention.

Despite the apparent success of ITNs in China, scientists and WHO officials did not assume that the intervention would necessarily work for malaria control in Africa. The idea that a single uniform technology could be used everywhere conflicted with a central dictum of malariologists in the post-eradication era. Vector control measures should be "appropriate" and tailored to specific vector biologies and ecologies.[29] East Asia and Africa had different malaria vectors with different characteristics, and malaria transmission was, in general, more intense in sub-Saharan Africa than in East Asia. Furthermore, China had already developed a well-functioning primary health care system through which to implement ITNs. Such systems did not exist in most malaria-endemic regions in Africa. Therefore, while China's experience partially inspired efforts to deploy the intervention on the continent, WHO officials and entomologists saw China as too incommensurate with Africa to be a valid testing ground for the new malaria control tool. For all their simplicity and seeming intuitiveness, ITNs did not scale up easily as a public health measure.

In the early 1980s, as China was beginning to incorporate ITNs into larger-scale public health programs, scientists working in West and East Africa initiated field trials with the technology to overcome this lack of transferability. They undertook these endeavors within prevailing intellectual and disciplinary frameworks in malaria research, which for decades had been dominated by entomology and a focus on mosquitoes.[30] They also did so in a political-economic context characterized by resource scarcity. These factors shaped scientists' research questions as they investigated the effects of ITNs on the continent.

There was certainly reason for scientists to doubt the technology's suitability for malaria control in Africa. In the late 1970s, entomologists investigating ordinary, untreated bed nets in The Gambia found that although nets greatly reduced mosquitoes' feeding success, they seemed to have little effect on malaria transmission in areas with highly efficient vectors, such as *Anopheles gambiae*, which could sustain transmission without feeding (or biting) very much.[31] This did not bode well because *Anopheles gambiae* were so predominant in sub-Saharan Africa. At this early stage, then, scientists and health officials viewed bed nets as, at best, a supplementary method and not one expected to shoulder much of the continent's malaria control burden.

But pyrethroids offered an extra punch, one that scientists thought could enhance the protection of a simple bed net. Entomologists from France's Office de la Recherche Scientifique et Technique Outre-Mer (Office of Scientific and Technical Research Overseas) contributed some of the first formal scientific investigations of ITNs on the continent, building on past experiences using insecticide-treated materials to control other insect vectors in West Africa. In 1983 Frédéric Derriet, Pierre Carnevale, and others used WHO funding to conduct an experimental hut trial with permethrin-treated nets in Burkina Faso. They concluded that nets impregnated with permethrin reduced man/vector contact to such a degree that, even when damaged, this tool "could become an effective method of malaria prevention for populations normally at risk of this disease."[32] British entomologists working in Tanzania, led by Chris Curtis from the London School of Hygiene and Tropical Medicine (LSHTM), also set up experimental hut trials to gauge the effect of ITNs on mosquito vectors. Around 1983, Curtis, his mentee Jo Lines, and colleagues from the Tropical Pesticides Research Institute in Arusha tested insecticidal curtains, bed nets, and anklets. Thinking pragmatically, they framed their results in terms of the suitability of insecticide-treated materials for community-run primary health care, which, when "organized locally . . . could avoid several of the problems encountered with centrally organized programmes of house spraying."[33] Like chloroquine, bed nets and insecticide solution could also be sold at local shops in places with no specially trained public health personnel. In other words, scientists were interested in ITNs not only for their physical and chemical properties but also for their feasibility in the political and economic context of rural Africa.

Although ITNs emerged as a potentially feasible solution to a simmering disease crisis in Africa, they by no means monopolized discussions of malaria vector control at this point. Members of the WHO Expert Committee on Vector Biology and Control recommended a wide variety of measures, including environmental management, larvivorous fish and other larvicides, and window screens. They did not abandon pesticide-spraying altogether, though they recommended it with much caution and felt most African countries did not have the resources to employ the method sustainably anyway.[34] ITNs did not stand out immediately or obviously as the best means of preventing malaria; if anything, they stood out as one of the more viable and tangible methods under prevailing resource constraints.

Scientists continued to conduct field studies with ITNs in East and Southeast Asia and the Western Pacific at this time, which seemed to reinforce optimism about the intervention.[35] Entomologists working in Africa cited experiences and studies from these places when amassing evidence for the effectiveness of ITNs. Again, the vector biologies and ecologies differed between the regions, so this evidence had a limited impact on assessments of the technology's effectiveness in Africa. Malaria experts did not understand ITNs as working equally well in all settings, even discounting operational factors such as the presence of an established primary health care program. This lack of generalizability deterred the WHO from recommending the tool widely for vector control.

Taking a Biomedical Turn

Understandings of insecticide-treated nets as medical objects that affected human disease indicators may seem inevitable. However, this conception has a history. Although entomologists in Africa had been testing the effects of insecticidal materials on mosquitoes—for example, on mosquito mortality and feeding rates—they were not examining the effects of these materials on human disease. The idea that ITNs could reduce one's risk of disease by blocking, repelling, or killing mosquitoes might seem obvious in retrospect. In the early 1980s, however, entomological evidence and gaps in knowledge about the relationship between infective mosquito bites and the manifestation of symptoms did not lead researchers to assume this. Instead, scientists with backgrounds and interests in human sciences working in specific contexts generated questions about the relationship between net use and symptomatic malaria illness. Measuring the protective, medical effects of ITNs on humans, rather than their effects on mosquitoes, these scientists began to redefine the tool in biomedical terms.

The British Medical Research Council (MRC) Laboratories in The Gambia—a narrow, 325-kilometer-long strip of land just south of the West African Sahel—served as an important origin point for bed nets' biomedical turn. The MRC had been doing research on malaria in the former British colony since 1948. Throughout the 1980s the MRC provided steady funding for its Gambian field stations to cover basic operation costs, which allowed researchers to establish and engage in long-term projects.[36] Few other research institutes on the continent were able to draw on this kind of support for malaria research at the time, given the relatively low political and financial interest in the disease.

Before 1980, much of the MRC's malaria research in The Gambia was entomological or parasitological, focusing on mosquitoes and parasites. Afterward, however, the institution's research profile began to shift toward studying malaria disease, especially among young children, for whom malaria was a considerable threat. This occurred after the MRC hired the physician Brian Greenwood to be director of the laboratories at the beginning of the decade. Greenwood had been working in Nigeria for fifteen years, moving into malaria and meningitis research by way of rheumatology.[37] Working in a context of limited scientific and medical resources, he sought to develop simple and practical methods of disease management. His background informed the types of research questions that the MRC investigated in The Gambia during the 1980s. These included seemingly simple ones such as how many children had died from or suffered a clinical episode of malaria in a year, which proved difficult to answer in a setting with limited health surveillance and record keeping.[38] Such questions framed malaria as a childhood disease (like measles) rather than a "tropical" parasitic and vector-borne disease, which called for medical rather than environmental management.

The WHO's promotion of primary health care also shaped the MRC's activities. Under Greenwood's direction, the MRC became involved in studying the impact of primary health care services on child mortality. These studies became part of the Gambian government's effort to set up primary health care services in villages. MRC scientists worked to integrate malaria control activities—at that time "fever management" and mass chemoprophylaxis with chloroquine—into these services.[39] With the threat of chloroquine resistance looming, Greenwood recognized the need to find alternative methods of malaria control.

Although ITNs were coming onto the scene as a possible alternative during the early 1980s, specific circumstances in The Gambia shaped the MRC's interest in testing this intervention. In preparation for primary health care activities in 1982, Greenwood and the demographer Andrew Bradley began to survey and map the area around Farafenni, a market town just south of the Senegalese border and home to one of the MRC's new field stations. They did a malaria morbidity survey in which, going from home to home, they noticed that many residents regularly used bed nets and canopies.[40] They attempted to measure the medical effects of nets by conducting a bed net survey, retrospectively correlating bed net use with lower splenomegaly (enlargement of the spleen) and parasitemia (the presence of malaria parasites in the blood) in young children.[41] Up to that point, malaria researchers had only collected anecdotal evidence suggesting that people who slept under nets had lower levels of parasitemia.[42] Of course, the MRC's new data did not bring closure and certainty. Were these lower levels of splenomegaly and parasitemia due to other factors, such as the location of people's homes or cultural practices associated with different ethnic groups? Unsure, Greenwood and Bradley felt their "findings need[ed] to be confirmed by intervention trials."[43] This is exactly what MRC scientists set out to do in the mid-1980s, hoping to elucidate the effects of bed nets on malaria disease in The Gambia.

The MRC's approach marked a subtle but important shift in the way people investigated bed nets as malaria control devices. Since the early twentieth century, health officials and malaria researchers had linked the control of mosquitoes to reductions in malaria cases. Scientists—primarily entomologists—tested bed nets and other vector control methods with this link in mind, typically measuring these methods' effects on mosquitoes to evaluate their public health potential. MRC scientists, by contrast, investigated bed nets'

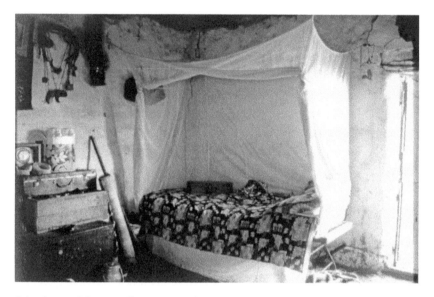

A bed net with entry flaps open, The Gambia, ca. 1990. Source: World Health Organization Image Library; photo by Steven Lindsay

effects on human disease outcomes. In doing so, they changed the indexes used to measure the success of this vector control tool from their effects on mosquitoes to their effects on humans. They also blended the domains of clinical medicine—traditionally concerned with the treatment of individual bodies—and public health—traditionally concerned with preventing disease among populations by ameliorating disease-promoting conditions.[44] This in turn allowed scientists to use experimental paradigms from biomedicine, such as randomized controlled trials, to test the efficacy of ITNs in subsequent years.

The MRC did not carry out additional bed net trials simply to produce scientific knowledge about the tool's medical efficacy; they also did so as part of the institution's larger commitment to test and develop primary health care in The Gambia. Following the Farafenni surveys, Greenwood and his colleagues initiated a three-year project on the effect of bed nets on malaria morbidity in children to, among other things, determine whether permethrin-treated bed nets "offer[ed] a practical approach to the control of malaria in African villages."[45] This work caught the eye of the Special Programme for Research and Training on Tropical Diseases (TDR), a multilateral program cosponsored by the WHO, World Bank, and United Nations Development Programme. TDR financed the development of cost-effective technologies to combat "tropical diseases" and, to a lesser extent, the building of research capacity in the countries most affected by these ailments. In this period the agency was also interested in mobilizing "community participation" to implement simple, effective, and sustainable health interventions, "a staple of WHO policy."[46] Its Applied Field Research in Malaria (FIELDMAL) working group, which focused on vector control, found ITNs potentially promising in this regard and funded the MRC's bed net trials with such priorities in mind.

The MRC conducted its first trial of ITNs in 1985 in Katchang, a rural village situated on the north bank of the River Gambia. Bob Snow, a young, eager doctoral student who came to run the new demographic surveillance site at Farafenni, conducted day-to-day operations alongside Gambian fieldworkers. The study enrolled nearly 400 participants who already used bed nets regularly, aiming to determine whether adding permethrin to those nets could reduce malaria morbidity in children under the age of ten. Greenwood and his colleagues designed the study as a randomized controlled trial, mimicking pharmaceutical trials. They even included a placebo arm, which used nets dipped in a dilute solution of crystal violet. They also used individual net users as the unit of analysis, based on the prevailing view that ITNs provided personal but not necessarily community-wide protection from malarious mosquitoes.[47]

Conducting a randomized controlled trial with ITNs, however, turned out to be much more complicated than doing so with pharmaceuticals. First, the research team carried out the experiment among a population using their own bed nets. This allowed investigators to save money on materials and time on educating study participants about how to hang bed nets. At the same time, this made the process of standardizing insecticide treatment more arduous. Snow had to determine how much water each type of net fiber absorbed to ensure that each net had the same dosage of insecticide, 0.5 grams per square meter. Residents also had different sizes of bed nets, which affected the amount of permethrin necessary to achieve this dosage.[48] Simply standardizing the intervention took considerable time and effort.

To make matters more complicated, neither the definition of a clinical attack of malaria nor the methods of malaria case detection had been standardized by this point.[49] Measuring malaria disease outcomes was especially difficult to do among such a large population and with limited laboratory resources. The symptoms of mild malaria illness, such as fever, sweating, chills, and headaches, are not wholly distinctive to malaria. One could not even confirm a malaria diagnosis based only on reported fever and an enlarged spleen. Snow and his team of fieldworkers tracked malaria morbidity by taking verbal autopsies and children's temperatures. They later confirmed parasitemia through blood work done at the labs in Farafenni, a task that itself can be difficult and time consuming.[50] By establishing methods for evaluating malaria disease indicators in rural villages and homesteads, as opposed to clinics, MRC scientists set the stage for subsequent bed net trials in Africa measuring the technology's effects on human disease.

Furthermore, Katchang residents came into the trial with their own understandings of bed nets, which did not necessarily match those of scientists. Members of the Mandinka ethnic group had long used bed nets to maintain conjugal privacy as well as protection from nuisance insects. Men often provided bed linen, including bed nets or canopies, as part of marital exchanges.[51] As Amy Patterson describes in her study of bed net use in south-central Mali, where men also commonly gave "marriage nets" to their wives, cultural taboos limited the sharing of nets within a household since bed nets were associated with beds and, by extension, sex.[52] Katchang residents also understood nets as objects meant for comfort, for example, providing warmth at night or keeping out pests, rather than as public health tools. For the most part, study participants in the Katchang trial used ITNs as scientists had intended. As in trials from other parts of the continent, however, participants' preexisting conceptions of bed nets and domestic practices sometimes affected who used the intervention, how and when they used it, and when they washed it in ways that impinged on scientific protocols.

Following the Katchang trial, the MRC branched out to other areas around Farafenni for their subsequent studies. Its work focused on villages where residents, primarily of the Fula ethnic group, did not use bed nets regularly. While Snow could standardize the intervention more easily since residents did not already own nets, he still depended heavily on local village authorities to control experimental conditions. Scientific work did not stop at taking temperatures, examining blood films, and conducting statistical analysis but entailed cultivating social relationships as well. "You build a rapport," Snow told me, "so you have people being compliant, they understand the studies. There's lots of village meetings that you have to have with the elders. You sit around a big baobab tree on what was called a *Bantaba*, which was sort of like a woven mesh on sticks. We would all sit round and say the opening of the Qur'an, so we'd feel settled. And then we'd begin our discussions on issues to do with the trial, or problems that the village was having."[53] The investigation and use of bed nets were highly localized practices—a fact scientists working on other trials would learn later.

It was essential for Snow and Gambian fieldworkers to engage with village residents and community authority structures because they needed to ensure that participants complied with sometimes opaque experimental practices to produce valid results. Study participants had to sleep under nets every day for the entire rainy season, when malaria transmission was highest, with nets properly tucked in to block mosquitoes. Scientists also needed blood samples from children to confirm the presence of parasites. Taking blood, understood as a vital and valuable life force, provoked some residents' suspicions of the MRC, and 20% of the participants ultimately refused to give blood samples in the final clinical survey.[54] Gathering data was a negotiating process in which people in the study area, including trial participants and village authorities, had the final say on what, if any, scientific knowledge researchers produced about ITNs.

Partway through its series of bed net trials, the MRC hired the entomologist Steve Lindsay to supplement data on malaria disease with data on mosquitoes. Overall, his results were quite positive: ITNs reduced mosquito biting by 83–92% compared to nets treated with a placebo solution of milk and water.[55] However, the study also confirmed that ITNs could not completely prevent mosquitoes from biting people, even if the nets reduced malaria infection and incidence among users. Parasitemia levels did not differ significantly between intervention and control villages by the end of the rainy season.[56] This, combined with the fact that ITNs seemed to be less effective in reducing malaria morbidity in high transmission areas of Burkina Faso and Papua New Guinea, led Snow and his colleagues to conclude that the intervention might be more useful in places with low or moderate malaria transmission.[57] Greenwood echoed this sentiment in his project report for TDR, adding, "Before permethrin-impregnated nets can be recommended for widespread use in Africa," scientists needed to "determine whether protection against malaria observed in The Gambia can be reproduced in other areas of Africa" where transmission was more intense and less seasonal.[58] ITNs seemed promising, but not as a generalizable solution to the problem of malaria in Africa.

This series of experiments underscored the contingency of the intervention's effects in other ways too. In 1986, for example, a plague of grasshoppers swarmed the country and ravaged crops following a period of heavy rains. The Gambian government wanted to spray insecticide to get rid of them, which, Greenwood feared, would reduce the mosquito population in the study area and make it more difficult to isolate the contribution of ITNs to reductions in malaria transmission.[59] The Gambian Department of Crop Protection Services agreed to avoid blanket aerial spraying and unnecessary spraying in the study area as much as possible to ensure that the project could continue. Study participants' preexisting ideas about cleanliness and care, particularly for luxury items such as bed nets, also led some to wash their nets more often than scientists had hoped, thus reducing the potency of the insecticide. Moreover, Lindsay and his colleagues theorized, residents of certain villages slept under their nets less regularly compared to residents of others because they observed fewer mosquitoes in their homes.[60] Various human and nonhuman factors affected whether and how ITNs worked as malaria control devices. Nets were not universal.

This lesson emerged in even greater detail from ethnographic work carried out during the trials. The anthropologist Carol MacCormack, who began working with the MRC in The Gambia in 1985, investigated social and cultural factors that affected bed net purchase and use, since these would affect the success of a future national bed net program. MacCormack surveyed residents to find out which net fabrics and colors they liked, how much they would be willing to pay for ITNs, and how cultural factors might influence their willingness to purchase nets. She reported, for instance, that nomadic and seminomadic Fula populations kept most of their wealth in cattle and preferred to have fewer goods around so they could more readily move with their herds. A preference for household goods over animals tended to fall along gender lines, with women expressing a greater interest in the former. Health programmers would need to choose net fabrics wisely, MacCormack emphasized, since some study participants thought certain fabrics "tore too easily to justify investment of D55" (around US$7 at the time).[61] The fabric had to hold up against the ragged sticks and millet stalks used for bed construction in many households. MacCormack also noted that since people's beds varied in size, "in an expanded programme[,] nets must be custom made by village tailors."[62] Of course, factors other than net quality—such as women bringing their infants out with them before dawn to pound millet or cook—could complicate a reliance on ITNs for malaria control.

Concerned with the practical aspects of using ITNs for public health, MRC scientists also produced knowledge about the suitability of nets for rural primary health care schemes. Snow and his colleagues, for example, published a paper on a new technique they used during one trial to treat large amounts of bed nets at once. This "dustbin technique," where one dipped many nets in a single, large drum of insecticide solution, they claimed, "provide[d] a practical method for impregnated bed nets suitable for use by [village health workers]." Previous methods, they felt, were "too complicated to be carried out by illiterate [village health workers] who would not be able to calculate the surface area of nets or to make appropriate concentrations of permethrin solution."[63] Given the success and speed of the dustbin technique, as well as the population's acceptance of sleeping under treated nets, investigators concluded that "insecticide-treated bed nets offer a potential method for malaria control that is well-suited to community participation and integration into a primary health care programme."[64] Pragmatic goals of finding simple, inexpensive tools that rural communities could implement themselves underpinned ITN research not just in The Gambia, but in Africa more generally.

Although early ITN trials in Africa highlighted the practical and public health utility of ITNs, the trials' findings did not translate into immediate adoption. In the late 1980s, WHO representatives convened a meeting in Geneva to discuss the ITN studies done up to that point. Most of these studies were small in scale, often comparing two villages with nets and two villages without nets. Incorporating sixteen villages, the MRC had done the largest bed net trials in Africa to date. And even though the Gambian trials had been randomized, they did not generate overwhelming evidence of the efficacy of ITNs in reducing malaria. Different research institutions had not coordinated their studies. Teams of investigators not only measured different outcomes, but they did not even measure some of these outcomes in the same way or test the same intervention. Some teams, for instance, tested insecticide-treated curtains hanging over people's windows. Scientists often distributed the ITNs to communities, but many of them measured the impact of the intervention on individual malaria sufferers, as if individuals were unaffected by the larger introduction of ITNs in the area.[65] As Lindsay recalled, the malaria epidemiologist Louis Molyneux "ripped everyone's studies to pieces" at that meeting.[66] Together these studies could not answer conclusively whether ITNs were effective for malaria control in Africa.

Becoming a Tool for Child Survival

As the early history of insecticide-treated net research makes clear, nothing about the life of this object was predetermined or straightforward. International health officials and malaria researchers were curious about using the technology to control malaria in rural Africa, but their initial scientific studies suggested that ITNs might have limited potential. Such feelings of promise and uncertainty infused the MRC's next bed net experiment. Proposed in 1988, it was the first experiment to test whether ITNs could reduce child mortality. In retrospect, this trial marked an important turning point in the life of ITNs, catalyzing its rise to global health fame. MRC investigators did not, however, foresee this outcome at the time. In fact, they only defined ITNs as tools for ensuring child survival as part of their ongoing, pragmatic efforts to test the intervention's suitability for primary health care in The Gambia.

Prevailing priorities in international health and development, along with the MRC's prior malaria research in The Gambia, informed this landmark experiment. In 1982 UNICEF launched the "Child Survival Revolution," aiming to bring simple, cheap technologies to low-income settings to reduce child mortality.[67] This helped focus attention on major childhood diseases, with malaria being one of the deadliest in rural sub-Saharan Africa. In addition, MRC scientists had already collected extensive data on bed nets and malaria in The Gambia. They had even developed techniques for measuring child mortality through postmortem questionnaires.[68] Greenwood and his team had also identified major causes of death among children in the region, giving them a substantial base of health data from which to measure the impact of ITNs on overall child mortality.[69]

Shifting knowledge and possibilities for malaria control in rural Africa made ITNs appear to be an increasingly desirable intervention. MRC investigators found that the treatment of presumptive episodes of malaria did not reduce child malaria mortality, even in areas where chloroquine was still effective. Cases of malaria turned fatal as quickly as two to three days after the onset of symptoms, Greenwood hypothesized, and it was very difficult for families to access drugs through volunteer health workers once they recognized a case of malaria.[70] Fear of increasing chloroquine resistance, combined with limited access to microscopy for diagnosis, compounded the difficulty of relying on treatment to curb malaria mortality. Preventive measures such as bed nets seemed much more valuable in helping children survive a bout of the disease.

Even given this increased attention to child survival, MRC researchers did not necessarily privilege questions about the effects of ITNs on child mortality from the outset. They continued to prioritize programmatic questions related to implementing the intervention through the country's vastly under-resourced primary health care system. Greenwood sent a research proposal for the trial to TDR's FIELDMAL group, the main funder of ITN projects in Africa by this point. The abbreviated list of objectives on the first page of this early proposal did not even mention mortality:

Objectives of Project

1. To determine whether village health workers (VHWs) can be taught to impregnate be [*sic*] nets safely and effectively with insecticide.
2. To determine whether targetted [*sic*] chemoprophylaxis combined with treated bed nets is more effective at reducing morbidity from malaria than treated bed nets alone.
3. To investigate community attitudes to chemoprophylaxis and treated bed nets as malaria control measures.[71]

MRC scientists initially foregrounded applied research outcomes for funders.

This project proposal illustrates that MRC scientists were already thinking about implementing ITNs when they designed the trial. Members of FIELDMAL encouraged Greenwood to include "community participation" and cost analyses as components of the trial, and gear it "towards continuity on a self-sustained basis" following the withdrawal of TDR support.[72] In line with suggestions from FIELDMAL, MRC investigators used this trial to assess whether the Gambian government could implement ITNs in a village-run primary health care system to reduce all-cause and malaria-specific mortality.[73] This experiment was not just an academic exercise to understand the impact of ITNs on disease; rather, it was part of a broader effort to build up rural health services and abate child death in a context of scarce resources.

An applied approach, of course, limited the replicability of this trial. The MRC team chose not to design the experiment as a randomized controlled trial—the gold standard for medical intervention trials. Instead, they monitored child morbidity and mortality among sixteen primary health care villages, where children received ITNs along with either the antimalarial drug Maloprim or a placebo drug. Scientists simultaneously monitored thirty-five smaller villages without primary health care services or village health workers, which received no interventions and served as controls. Although scientists recognized that research questions "could have been answered more satisfactorily by a randomised control trial," this would mean that one group of children would receive both placebo tablets and placebo-dipped nets.[74] Since previous studies showed that both interventions could help prevent malaria, scientists argued that it would be unethical to deny one group the interventions. The MRC had to balance scientific standards and protocols with realities of health care in The Gambia.

The MRC research team continued to investigate whether village health workers could adequately dose bed nets with insecticide, hoping that these workers could eventually take over the practice once the experiment ended. Women's groups and "traditional birth attendants" helped health workers measure out permethrin in wash bins stationed at village centers. Mothers would dip their nets in the insecticide and then lay the nets to dry on mattresses at home. While practical from the point of view of a health program, this process was imperfect for standardizing an experimental intervention. MRC scientists discovered that the concentration of permethrin varied between bed nets, attributing this to possible spillage of insecticide during the treatment process, insecticide dripping off the nets when women took them home, or insecticide dripping off during the drying phase.[75] This dilemma did not nullify results, though it did reveal just how complicated it could be to assemble this malaria control technology in practice.

During the early months of the trial, the findings on child mortality did not look particularly promising. As Lindsay recalled, one of the clinicians working in the region had collected data suggesting that nets were not having much effect. "We thought, 'oh well. That was it.'"[76] However, the epidemiologist and principal investigator on the trial, Pedro Alonso, continued plotting mortality data. By the end of the trial's first year, October 1989, he reported incredible results. Mortality rates in intervention villages had decreased dramatically for children one- to four years old, even among those taking the placebo drug. This was not only the case for malaria-specific mortality but also for deaths from all causes. Alonso produced a histogram com-

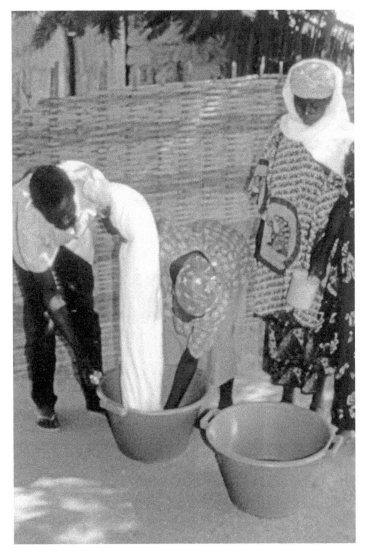

Dipping a bed net in insecticide, The Gambia, ca. 1990. Source: World Health Organization Image Library; photo by Steven Lindsay

paring all-cause mortality among the intervention and control groups. The graph for the intervention group showed an initial peak in mortality in October 1988, before the intervention period commenced, followed by a rapid and sustained drop extending into June 1990. Mortality levels in this group had been, in Lindsay's words, "decapitated."[77] The graph for the control group, on the other hand, had two, consistent mortality peaks marking the end of the rainy seasons—one in October 1988, one in October 1989.[78] Calculating the difference in mortality rates between the two groups, investigators found the intervention (ITNs plus either Maloprim or a placebo) had a protective efficacy of 63%.[79] This statistic, combined with the histogram, provided a powerful visual argument for ITNs.

The variability and contingencies of experimental conditions nevertheless led the MRC to qualify its findings and the applicability of results. The region experienced much less rainfall in 1990, and thus lower malaria transmission and rates of overall mortality as well. The group that received an ITN and Maloprim experienced notable reductions in mortality over the course of the year, but mortality rates for the ITN/placebo group came out roughly the same as those for the control group—both fairly low. Based on data from 1990, then, ITNs by themselves appeared to have little impact on child mortality when malaria transmission and mortality were already very low.

Alonso and the rest of the MRC research team were unsure whether the similarity between mortality rates in controls and the ITN/placebo arm was some "statistical quirk" due to fewer overall deaths in 1990, or whether chemoprophylaxis with Maloprim enhanced protection from deadly malaria parasites or other microorganisms. Therefore, Greenwood reported to TDR, "the results of the 1990 study illustrate the way in which the effects of impregnated bed nets on mortality and morbidity from malaria are influenced by the level of malaria transmission in the community in which they are used." This "emphasise[d] the need for further studies of impregnated bed nets in areas of varying malaria transmission before their true potential as a malaria control measure can be ascertained."[80] Alonso and colleagues underscored this issue of local variability in their published results, reporting that "the importance of malaria as a cause of death, the nature and habits of the dominant malaria vector, and the acceptance of bed nets are all factors which vary from area to area and which may affect the efficacy of this intervention."[81] The MRC's mortality trial reinforced findings from earlier studies showing that ITNs could have a different impact due to numerous local circumstances.

Nevertheless, their findings from the first year of the trial were remarkable. And since child mortality declined among both Maloprim and placebo groups, scientists linked the reductions to one tool primarily: the ITN. Their findings on all-cause mortality also suggested that preventing malaria could help prevent other leading causes of child death, though they did not have a clear explanation for this. However, they did not need to describe the exact mechanism by which the technology reduced child mortality—an indicator for which it can be difficult to attribute a single or direct cause. The statistics seemed to say it all. MRC scientists, along with Gambian research assistants, study participants, village health workers, and village authorities, refashioned a mundane vector control technology into a tool for ensuring child survival—an outcome many in the policy sphere considered a "benchmark of public health impact."[82] This significantly raised the profile of ITNs as a potential means of mitigating Africa's growing malaria crisis.

While many people identified the MRC's mortality trial as a turning point, scientists, health officials, and donors varied in their responses to its results. Jo Lines, who had been investigating insecticidal materials in Tanzania since the early 1980s, thought scientists had shown that ITNs were effective for malaria control by the early 1990s. It was time to "let the world invest."[83] Steve Lindsay felt similarly, telling me, "I thought, 'publish this paper in the *Lancet*, you've got these papers out, gone to WHO, bish, bash, bosh—job done. Take it away boys. Scale up.'"[84] Indeed, he recalled, some people reacted to the finding as if it were obvious—"My grandmother could have told you that!"[85] Some organizations, such as UNICEF and the African Medical and Research Foundation, had even started distributing ITNs on a small scale around this time, as chapter 3 documents in greater detail.

Many, however, did not think this finding about ITNs was obvious, nor were they completely convinced by the MRC's mortality trial. This included some consultants at WHO headquarters who did not feel that the experiment substantiated the large-scale implementation of ITN programs in Africa.[86] This and previous bed net experiments were simply too individual, too singular in their results, they argued, to extrapolate scientific findings. The Swiss epidemiologist and coordinator of subsequent bed net trials, Christian Lengeler, remembered that the results from The Gambia trial were exciting, but "people were a bit cautious about the result" because the trial had not been "sufficiently randomized."[87] Since the long-term effects of ITNs remained uncertain, WHO officials also feared that the intervention just diverted mosquitoes to people without nets and reduced malaria immunity among net users, a phenomenon that could lead to spikes in malaria deaths once people stopped using control measures.[88]

In the face of this hesitancy, ITN activities did not extend much beyond a few small programs, often run by research agencies or nongovernmental organizations (NGOs) in conjunction with African health officials. The WHO's Malaria Control Department had little money to invest in bed nets. TDR had more interest in and capacity to do so, but the organization funded scientific research and training, not health programs. Thinking that African communities might value and purchase bed nets for "privacy and protection from nuisance insects," the WHO Expert Committee on Malaria did see an opportunity to foster inexpensive, decentralized malaria control through this technology. Yet, in 1992, they continued to promote chemoprophylaxis alongside a range of mosquito prevention measures, leaving large-scale bed net programs for the future.[89] Although a few organizations and African governments were disseminating ITNs in the early 1990s, the technology remained marginal in the international malaria control tool kit.

Demonstrating the Value of ITNs in Africa

While some experts did not embrace insecticide-treated nets in the early 1990s, TDR and its director, Tore Godal, found the intervention promising. Godal, a Norwegian physician who specialized in microbiology and immunology, took over the directorship of TDR in 1986. Seeking to overcome negative critiques of ITN research, he decided to sponsor a series of randomized controlled trials in different field sites across Africa. He hoped these experiments could produce definitive scientific proof that ITNs reduced child mortality outside The Gambia, including in areas of moderate or high malaria transmission.[90] Godal, who had a history of defying WHO opposition in order to test out new medical interventions, put about half of TDR's budget behind testing nets.[91] As Lengeler recalled, he "basically stopped a lot of other projects just to finance the bed net trials."[92] Godal also set up a Taskforce on Bed Nets, which replaced FIELDMAL, to oversee the organization's new "Bed Net Initiative."

Godal's decision to sponsor a multisite study of ITNs fit within a growing trend of using randomized controlled trials in international health. Over the 1980s, donor criticisms concerning the lack of accountability in aid spending as well as reformers' desires to make the field more scientifically rigorous and better able to manage variability between contexts spurred calls for greater quantification and experimentation in international health. The growing emphasis on pharmaceutical interventions further contributed to

policy makers' appeals for randomized controlled trial evidence.[93] The experiments at the heart of TDR's Bed Net Initiative actually represented an early
example of using large-scale randomized controlled trials to test nonpharmaceutical and nonvaccine interventions, the other being trials of vitamin A
supplementation.[94] Since it was difficult to demonstrate that vitamin A or
ITNs alone caused reductions in child mortality—the mechanism of action
being unclear—one needed to show reductions among thousands of people
to claim that the correlations did not happen by chance. In figuring out how
to design these experiments of vitamin A supplementation and ITNs in the
1980s and 1990s, research teams helped lay the groundwork for subsequent
randomized controlled trials testing nonpharmaceutical health and development interventions.

The Taskforce on Bed Nets helped set up these trials as demonstrations
of value in multiple senses. Based on the randomized controlled trial paradigm, these trials were supposed to demonstrate the value of ITNs in saving
children's lives through the language of clinical epidemiology and biostatistics. Measuring the cost-effectiveness of ITNs, health economists aimed to
demonstrate the value of the intervention in relieving financial burdens on
ailing health systems, as well as the value potential donors would receive by
investing in nets to save lives. Incorporating community education into experiments, investigators sought to demonstrate the value of ITNs as public
health measures to study participants. Just as in The Gambia, however, the
experiments also illustrated the contingency of the evidence supporting the
intervention's efficacy.

The epidemiologist Jacqueline Cattani, who managed the Taskforce on
Bed Nets, selected four sites for ITN trials at the group's April 1992 meeting.
These included the entire country of The Gambia (scaling up the MRC's
original mortality trial); Navrongo, in northeastern Ghana; Kilifi, on the
Kenyan coast; and Oubritenga, in central Burkina Faso. She and her committee members considered these as ideal test sites because they already contained some existing research infrastructure, including medical research
institutes and networks of village health workers. Investigators had already
collected or inherited some health and demographic data from previous
projects in these places.[95] The research institutions that would be running
the trials, moreover, had ties with their respective countries' ministries of
health. That relationship was important to TDR because its officials wanted
scientific results to inform national programs and policies at the end of the

experiments.[96] Finally, all the sites represented different "epidemiological settings" with different levels and types of malaria transmission, ranging from low seasonal transmission in The Gambia to high seasonal transmission in Burkina Faso.

To ensure comparability of experiment results, Christian Lengeler, then at the LSHTM, came onto the project as the "Bednet Coordinator." Coordinating the experiments from London, he helped standardize experimental methods, materials, and outcomes measured across the four field trials. At the same time, each experiment also incorporated some unique element that would contribute new knowledge about ITNs. The trial in The Gambia, for example, would measure the effectiveness of ITNs in the context of the country's new National Bednet Programme, established in 1992. The Burkina Faso trial tested curtains rather than bed nets because, as investigators noted, people in the study area did not live in houses big enough to accommodate bed nets easily and could not afford bed nets in the first place.[97] Because they had established a district hospital surveillance system that tracked severe, life-threatening malaria among children, the team in Kilifi set out to measure the effect of ITNs on rates of severe malaria.[98] Local circumstances shaped study design.

At their core, all four experiments sought to evaluate two things: the efficacy of ITNs in reducing mortality among children twelve- to fifty-nine months old and the cost-effectiveness of ITNs in the research site. The first objective functioned as an extension of the MRC's original mortality trial in The Gambia; policy makers and scientists wanted to confirm that ITNs could reduce child mortality in places with higher malaria transmission pressure. Moreover, scientists still did not know exactly how ITNs reduced mortality. Therefore, it was crucial that the new experiments demonstrate statistically that ITNs had a consistent protective effect across contexts. Only then would members of the international health and development community accept ITNs as scientifically validated, widely applicable interventions.

All four trials also measured the cost-effectiveness of ITNs. Health economists considered this information important since resources, especially for malaria control, remained tight. Anne Mills, a health economist from the LSHTM, acted as Lengeler's counterpart for this aspect of the study, establishing formulas for economists from each trial to use in their evaluations.[99] She had measured cost-effectiveness for the original mortality trial in The Gambia as well, finding that "for the first time a malaria control strategy in

Africa has been shown to be competitive with other interventions that pre-vent child deaths."[100] If researchers could demonstrate scientifically that ITNs were cost-effective and could reduce child mortality (i.e., in a way that could be reproduced and achieve the same general result), this tool could be a viable candidate for scarce health and development resources.

The research teams of all four TDR-sponsored trials also included evalu-ations of community attitudes, perceptions, and acceptance of bed nets as a research objective to establish the feasibility of introducing ITNs into these regions. What African populations thought about ITNs was critical because, as scientists and program planners believed, residents of malaria-endemic areas would not only have to use the intervention but pay for it as well.[101] Moreover, health officials were well aware that malaria eradication activities faltered in the past because DDT-spray teams did not coordinate with or ac-commodate local populations.[102] Every research team had an applied an-thropologist or other social scientist who issued questionnaires and con-ducted focus group discussions with study participants. In reporting their results, investigators emphasized that most participants wanted bed nets and insecticide treatment but often could not afford these products.[103] Social scientists also found that most people did not believe that mosquitoes were the cause or the sole cause of malaria. They more often desired nets because the devices protected against nuisance insects.[104] Qualitative research into whether communities would adopt ITNs, even despite a lack of famil-iarity with the technology, served broader goals of teaching people that they should value and desire the intervention.[105]

Beyond these surveys, investigators did various things to prepare com-munities for the introduction of an ITN experiment. A couple of research teams set up different "culturally specific" channels for disseminating edu-cational messages about bed nets. The team from the Kenya Medical Re-search Institute and Wellcome Trust in Kilifi organized poster competitions, youth-group theater performances, and *barazas* (community meetings) to disseminate messages about the benefits of ITNs and their proper use.[106] In Burkina Faso, the Centre National de Lutte contre le Paludisme team organized Burkinabe traditional theater performances, poster competitions, and village-wide "causerie-débats" for the same purpose.[107] In the context of The Gambia's national bed net program, the MRC and Gambian Ministry of Health used radio shows and T-shirts illustrating correct dipping proce-dures to inform people about re-treating their nets with insecticide.[108] Such activities were important to ensuring compliance and generating sound scientific results.

Personnel who carried out mortality surveys, helped dose the bed nets with insecticide, and disseminated messages to study participants were crucial to the demonstrative goals of these trials as well. Some research teams benefited from having personnel in the region who could act as community liaisons or health workers. The Navrongo team, for example, inherited quite a lot of field research infrastructure from the Ghana Vitamin A Supplementation Trial project, including village key informants trained to collect demographic information from households.[109] The Kilifi team seconded public health officers and public health technicians from Kenya's Ministry of Health to act as community educators during the trial, in part to "ensure sustainability of the intervention at the end of the trial."[110] The Kilifi team also set up local bed net committees through Kenya's fledgling primary health care scheme to resolve participants' issues with bed nets. These intermediaries were critical in collecting data from and ensuring compliance of thousands of study participants, enough to produce statistically valid results. They were additionally important for demonstrating that ITNs could theoretically fit into existing community-run health infrastructure across rural Africa, which was still sparse or ad hoc in many places.

Despite scientists' well-planned, well-organized efforts, various obstacles threatened the trials. Sometimes the requirements of randomized controlled trials presented the obstacle. In Kilifi, scientists found that child mortality rates were much lower than expected. Therefore, they might have to increase the sample size or prolong the trial to achieve statistically significant results. They deemed both options infeasible since the control group was already complaining about not receiving nets and TDR funds were running low.[111] Furthermore, HIV prevalence among children in Kilifi was high—roughly 23%—which made it difficult to predict the "true effects of a malaria-specific intervention [on child mortality]." Bob Snow, who had left The Gambia for the Kenyan coast, initially planned to defer to the study's second objective (defining the impact of ITNs on severe malaria), fearing they would not have statistically robust findings on reductions in child mortality.[112]

In another instance, MRC scientists found that ITNs did not demonstrate protective effects in one of the five zones evaluated in its effectiveness trial. In reporting results back to TDR, Brian Greenwood attributed this to noncompliance among villagers in that area, emphasizing that ITNs showed a strong protective effect in the other four zones.[113] Investigators in Burkina Faso encountered a similar problem, finding that insecticide-treated curtains appeared to reduce child mortality in the first year of the trial but had no effect in the second year—a year when child mortality in the control group was inexplicably low.[114] Even with these hiccups, investigators had the statistical data to argue that on the whole, taking into account all groups and all years of the trials, ITNs were efficacious in reducing child mortality in all of these sites. The fact that they could demonstrate this despite noncompliance and anomalous mortality patterns, they claimed, just meant that findings underestimated the "true effects" of ITNs on child mortality.[115]

Many of the trials also suffered from financial woes. In both Kilifi and Burkina Faso, governments had devalued the currency as part of IMF and World Bank structural adjustment policies. This occurred after research institutions had received grant money for the year and converted it into local currency. In Kilifi, inflation was so high that the research team's estimated expenses for fuel costs alone rose by US$15,000 for the year.[116] TDR was unable to provide money to the Navrongo study to purchase bed nets and insecticide in its second year. Principal Investigator Fred Binka had to ask UNICEF and other organizations to procure these fundamental items instead. Ultimately, the Navrongo team could not even secure enough insecticide to re-treat all the nets in the intervention arm of the study. Mistakenly assuming that TDR would provide funding for insecticide, MRC researchers also had to cobble together donations from UNICEF, Action Aid, and other NGOs to carry out their national program.[117] Multiple teams had problems with timely or complete delivery of nets to study sites, which interfered with experimental protocols.[118]

These difficulties in coordinating large ITN trials foreshadowed logistical difficulties in running large-scale bed net programs in Africa, difficulties that seemed especially relevant insofar as most African governments would have to import both nets and insecticide. These complications also indicate a broader issue in global public health: policy makers assume that heavily funded, carefully monitored trials offer proof of concept—for example, that interventions such as ITNs reduce child mortality—but they often overlook the fact that trial conditions cannot be replicated in practice. Without reliable supply chains or funding streams, health officials might not even be able to acquire necessary resources for bed net programs, much less monitor and promote the use of the intervention. Scientists downplayed the issues with funding in their published results, which, as was standard, focused on the protective efficacy and cost-effectiveness findings.

Despite the challenges of conducting randomized controlled trials with ITNs, experimental findings seemed positive. At their least protective, ITNs (or insecticide-treated curtains, rather) reduced child mortality in Burkina Faso by 15%.[119] At their most protective, they reduced child mortality by 33% in Kilifi—just enough to demonstrate statistical significance there.[120] Together, these trials appeared to demonstrate how critical malaria control was to child survival in Africa by the simple fact that a malaria-specific intervention could reduce child mortality to such a significant degree.[121] While also exciting, calculations showing that ITNs were extremely cost-effective and survey findings indicating that people desired the intervention sat uneasily alongside the recognition that those most at risk for malaria would not be able to afford them.[122] Nonetheless, for health officials seeking to attract the support of major aid agencies, ITNs and malaria control more generally finally began to seem like a good investment.

ITNs came of age during a period of retraction, rethinking, and pessimism as the failure of existing malaria control methods and a global economic crisis exacerbated malaria in Africa. Nets represented one of the few feasible possibilities for curbing this disease on the continent under prevailing conditions of resource scarcity. Beginning in the 1980s, scientists worked with local health workers, village authorities, and residents from African research sites to produce scientific knowledge about nets, often with the hope of incorporating the intervention into inchoate primary health care programs. Through this research, especially that from The Gambia, ITNs and malaria were increasingly defined in biomedical terms. Furthermore, as scientists discovered, multiple contingencies—from global supply chains, to concurrent disease epidemics, to fluctuating rainfall levels, to people's use of ITNs—all affected whether and how the intervention saved lives.

When research teams conducted a series of large-scale randomized controlled trials over the mid-1990s, these contingencies did not disappear. However, the statistical nature of the experimental paradigm allowed investigators to render such factors as anomalies or potential confounders, or simply omit them altogether. ITNs' ability to save children's lives in a cost-effective way and within weak, decentralized health systems became the distillate abstracted from these experiments. These trials, then, did not just place Africa at the center of global health knowledge production; they also crystallized ITNs as politically valent, economically viable, and scientifically validated tools worthy of financial investment. As new quantification and experimental practices of evidence-based public health promised to objectively adjudicate scarce health resources, ITNs emerged as the "right tool for the job."[123]

2

The Biomedical Technology

From Kenyan Particulars to Global Universals

I met Michael Onyango on a warm December day in 2015. He was waiting for me at Kalandin Junction, about three kilometers north of the shores of Asembo Bay. We chatted about his life in this small dusty corner of western Kenya as we made the short trek to his house. Onyango said people in the area knew him as a "CDC guy," a title bestowed on him for his many years working on research projects with the US Centers for Disease Control and Prevention (CDC). After beginning as a mosquito collector in the mid-1980s, Onyango worked his way up to become a field coordinator on the largest-ever efficacy trial of insecticide-treated nets a decade later. He recounted his experience from that trial, his children looking on from the couch. He sounded particularly proud of his efforts to educate fellow Asembo residents about bed nets, malaria, and the goals of what for many was a puzzling endeavor. After the trial ended, he went around with some of the scientists to *barazas* (community meetings) in participating villages to announce the results. "Many of them were happy" to hear that bed nets saved children's lives, which, in the context of the region's HIV/AIDS and malaria crises, was more than welcome news. "I remember one time," he continued, "Dr. Bernard [Nahlen] was telling them, now if you take your children to the hospital, you get a vaccine, maybe for [an]other illness. These vaccines never came from heaven. Someone, some people, volunteered to participate in the study. And now that study is benefiting everybody. . . . It was just like we are in Asembo here; you have agreed to participate in this bed net project. So everybody in Kenya or in the world where malaria is a problem will benefit because you all volunteered to participate in this study."[1] Onyango's neighbors' trust in him helped transform a seeming matter of faith into a matter of scientific reason.

This randomized controlled trial capped off a series of experiments in the 1990s testing whether ITNs could reduce child mortality in Africa. While research teams had initiated efficacy trials with the intervention in areas with seasonal malaria transmission by 1994, no one had done so in an area of intense, year-round transmission. Thus, in 1996 scientists from the CDC and Kenya Medical Research Institute (KEMRI) set out to prove that ITNs could reduce child mortality even under the most extreme conditions of malaria and poverty, which characterized Onyango's hometown at the time. This goal of demonstrating that ITNs worked as universally applicable biomedical technologies capable of saving lives the same way everywhere was embedded in the experiment's design and scientists' framing of their statistical findings.

Even though scientists privileged the generalizable, or global, biomedical value of ITNs, they still had to demonstrate this value somewhere; that somewhere was Kenya's Siaya district (which includes the administrative location of Asembo).[2] As Onyango's memories of his work as a "CDC guy" underscore, the production of seemingly universal biomedical knowledge is an act heavily rooted in specificity; it involves specific research sites with specific researchers measuring specific outcomes among specific people. In global health, such an achievement vitally depends on the work of people like Onyango and his neighbors, who not only incorporate experimental interventions into their lives but also are able to convince others to do so. Global health science rests on their efforts as much as it does on claims that a health intervention works the same way everywhere, regardless of local contingencies. By generalizing—or, as Vincanne Adams terms it, "scaling up"—local claims about the efficacy of ITNs in Siaya into global health knowledge, scientists defined these objects as universally applicable biomedical technologies.[3]

Expanding on insights from chapter 1, this chapter examines in-depth how ITNs became consolidated as lifesaving biomedical tools. It does so through a historical ethnography of the KEMRI and CDC's (hereafter KEMRI-CDC) major ITN trial in Siaya.[4] Interweaving archival and published material with oral histories, the chapter interrogates how various groups—including Kenyan scientists, *nyamrerwa* (community health workers), their supervisors, and study participants—shaped the production of biomedical knowledge about this object.[5] Through their intellectual and material practices, and using their scientific, technical, and social skills, they helped generate local and specific claims about the efficacy of nets in Siaya. Expatriate scientists who designed research protocols depended heavily on the work of these various groups, even though not all parties shared the same understanding of malaria, bed nets, or research. Similarly, the landscape of Siaya—its environment, its residents, and residents' social relations—shaped the knowledge that scientists could produce about ITNs and how they produced it.[6] The history and circumstances of Siaya were not incidental to the production of universal biomedical knowledge; they were some of its critical building blocks.

When scientists circulated their findings from the experiment in publications, generalizing these results as global health knowledge, they stripped away details about how much and what kind of labor it took to get ITNs to save lives in Siaya. Statistics about how many lives nets saved or the number of hospital visits they prevented received top billing, since these data carried more value than local contingencies in the enterprise of global health. This was especially so because the Siaya experiment was meant to fill in open questions left by earlier trials sponsored by the Special Programme for Research and Training in Tropical Diseases (TDR) (described in chapter 1) and to confirm for policy makers and donors that ITNs would work anywhere. Siaya essentially served as a proxy for places with intense malaria transmission. Scientists did not ignore how the specific context of the region shaped the way they carried out the experiment. But in presenting this context as a backdrop to the knowledge production process rather than as an integral part of it, they dissociated ITN technology from the factors necessary to its function as a malaria control tool, such as users' sleeping habits or decisions to re-treat nets with insecticide. The lessons that scientists learned about the challenges of using this seemingly simple tool to save lives in Siaya did not travel along with efficacy statistics. The identity that ITNs acquired as a biomedical technology, then, was a precarious one, pieced together at the intersection of different epistemologies and at different scales of intervention by the scientific language and conventions of evidence-based public health.

Laying the Foundations of the ITN Trial in Siaya

As with other African centers of medical knowledge production, Siaya's social, political, ecological, and epidemiological history shaped its emergence as a major site of global health research.[7] Scientists had conducted malaria research in what was formerly Nyanza Province (Siaya's larger administrative home) beginning in the colonial period. The region's proximity to Lake Victoria and the equatorial climate fostered large populations of malaria-carrying mosquitoes. Irrigation schemes for cultivating sugarcane, and later rice, further promoted malaria transmission. In addition, neither the colonial government nor the post-independence Kenyan government invested substantially in this politically marginalized region populated predominantly by members of the Luo ethnic group. Impoverished living conditions and a dearth of health infrastructure exacerbated malaria, making Nyanza a fruitful place to study the disease.

This focus on malaria persisted as Kenyan officials founded new scientific and medical research institutions during the late 1970s and early 1980s.[8] Shortly after its establishment in 1979, KEMRI absorbed the Malaria and Other Protozoal Diseases Research Centre, located in Nyanza's provincial capital of Kisumu. Although the center had little in the way of laboratory equipment or staff, KEMRI's leadership felt it was well placed to study diseases affecting rural areas, "in which about 90% of the population of Kenya share, work, and live."[9] Rising rates of chloroquine resistance after 1980 attracted researchers seeking new ways to address malaria with diminishing financial and therapeutic resources, not only through new drug distribution schemes but also via the development of "economically feasible diagnostic tools" for rural health units.[10] This work augmented that of Kenya's Division of Vector-Borne Diseases, an arm of the Ministry of Health, which carried out malaria control activities and had its own laboratories in Kisumu.

To increase its presence overseas, the CDC also helped expand malaria research in Nyanza around this time. Harrison Spencer of the CDC's Division of Parasitic Diseases, an early conduit for this work, set up a field station in Nairobi in 1979. The following year he joined his colleague Dan Kaseje, a professor of community medicine at the University of Nairobi, on a chloroquine distribution project in Kaseje's home village of Saradidi, in Siaya.[11] In the process, they set up a network of village health workers who continued to work on subsequent research projects. Their investigations not only attracted international attention among the malaria control community but also fostered greater collaboration between CDC and Kenyan scientists in the region. In 1984 the CDC established a field station in Kisian on the outskirts of Kisumu, partnering with what was then renamed the KEMRI Vector Biology and Control Research Centre (VBCRC).[12] The center focused heavily on malaria in rural areas—and Siaya in particular—prioritizing the local application of research findings.

While KEMRI and CDC scientists working with the VBCRC did many studies on the issue of chloroquine resistance, they also spent considerable time investigating malaria vectors. When ITNs emerged as a potential vector control measure and alternative to drug-based approaches, Kenyan entomologists and their CDC colleagues joined the investigation of the intervention. They conducted a trial of permethrin-treated bed nets and curtains in Uriri (in Siaya) in 1988. This was the first trial to demonstrate that insecticidal curtains—fabric draped to cover a house's windows, doors, and eaves—were comparably effective to treated bed nets and, they concluded, "have a place in malaria control."[13] Since curtains required less netting material and insecticide per household than did personal-use bed nets, scientists considered it important to prove that this cheaper alternative had public health value. Two years later, a new cohort of entomologists conducted a second trial in Uriri to determine whether these interventions worked as well during seasons of very high malaria transmission.[14]

These scientists continued testing insecticide-treated materials during the early 1990s with an eye toward feasibility and sustainability. The VBCRC's director, Aggrey Oloo, led a research project in Kisumu, dubbed the Sisal Strands Project, which investigated the efficacy of curtains and bed nets made from the plentiful homegrown fiber, sisal.[15] This research, sponsored by TDR, aimed to find inexpensive, locally sourced malaria interventions suitable for the impoverished area. African scientists elsewhere proposed similar innovations around this time, such as insecticide-treated wall cloths and nets targeted to certain areas of the body, knowing that any malaria control activities would have to be done cheaply.[16] They also recognized that in some places people might not accept bed nets because they found them inconvenient, did not understand their importance, or did not have houses or sleeping spaces that easily accommodated the bed net design.[17] The Sisal Strands Project ultimately shut down around 1992, as TDR moved much of its funding into large-scale randomized controlled trials with ITNs (the "Bed Net Initiative" described in chapter 1). The project's fate highlights how TDR's twin aims of fostering research self-sufficiency in low-income countries and developing low-cost disease control tools aligned in some ways but not others.[18]

As the VBCRC expanded and churned out more internationally recognized malaria research over the late 1980s and early 1990s, it became involved in a new line of inquiry: malaria vaccine development. Malaria vaccines attracted the attention of those seeking to address malaria in Africa as well as to protect the militaries of industrialized countries. In this way, malaria vaccine research was more outward facing in its orientation than much of the center's other malaria work, which was aimed at informing Kenya's public health activities. KEMRI-CDC's initial forays into vaccine-related studies in Siaya played a direct role in the district becoming the site of a major randomized controlled trial with ITNs in the mid-1990s—a similarly outward-facing research project.

KEMRI-CDC's vaccine-related research began in earnest in 1992 with the initiation of the Asembo Bay Cohort Project. This study, located in and around the lakeside village of Asembo Bay, investigated the relationship between malaria infection and symptomatic disease in the hope of understanding how children acquired immunity to malaria. The research team used household demographic surveillance with community health workers to follow 1,848 pairs of mothers and their children in 15 villages. They sought to characterize factors associated with the acquisition of malaria infection, understand how malaria infection progressed to illness, and determine how people with little to no malaria immunity acquired it under "natural conditions."[19] In other words, scientists asked, how and why do children around Asembo Bay become infected with malaria, and why does that infection manifest as certain symptoms over time? The answers to these questions would provide important insights for the development of a malaria vaccine that might not be able to prevent infection completely but could potentially keep an infection from turning into life-threatening illness.

The Asembo Bay Cohort Project had another main goal, which acknowledged the area's socioeconomic realities but in a different way from earlier applied malaria control research. "Barring the massive improvements in standards of living or access to high-quality health care," CDC scientists wrote, "large-scale community-based interventions that either prevent infection, reduce the rate or intensity of exposure, or attenuate the clinical progression to severe disease are most likely the only interventions that will have a significant impact in the foreseeable future. . . . A reliable assessment of the intervention's efficacy . . . requires an extensive and thorough understanding of the dynamics and natural history of malaria infection and disease in the area in which they are tested."[20] The Asembo Bay Cohort Project was supposed to provide foundational knowledge necessary to test malaria control interventions in Siaya, though not necessarily interventions that were economically attainable for the population. Equipped with health and demographic data and a network of community health workers, scientists conducting the study helped fashion Siaya into a representative test site for malaria control in rural, resource-poor Africa—a perfect place to investigate ITNs.

Making Global Public Goods in Siaya

Indeed, Siaya became the place where scientists filled in many remaining gaps in knowledge about the efficacy of insecticide-treated nets on the continent. The district represented both an impoverished rural area of malaria-endemic Africa and a site of intense year-round malaria transmission. The CDC scientists who designed the randomized controlled bed net trial in Siaya aimed to produce knowledge that could contribute to malaria control in Kenya. Unlike with the Sisal Strands Project, however, they designed this experiment in such a way as to generate scientific knowledge that would be considered a "global public good." They wanted to produce something that could be "useful everywhere in the world, in every local context," not just western Kenya.[21] The experiment's design, infused with this goal of producing a global public good, ultimately circumscribed the information that scientists paid attention to during the trial and the ways in which they did so.

Although the CDC was building on work conducted under TDR's Bed Net Initiative, it largely operated under a different funding stream. The CDC drew on resources from the US government, specifically the United States Agency for International Development (USAID), for the experiment. This marked a shift in US funding for malaria, which since the 1970s had been directed mainly toward finding a malaria vaccine and alternative antimalarial drugs capable of protecting American military personnel overseas. This changed in the early 1990s when President George H. W. Bush called for the United States to get more involved in improving child survival in Africa.[22] In response, USAID created a new mechanism to increase the use of research, analysis, and information in support of better health policies and programs on the continent. As part of this, USAID provided $1 million to the CDC to conduct the ITN trial in Siaya—the largest sum any research team had received to conduct a bed net trial in Africa. Prioritizing the production of universally applicable, generalizable knowledge, the agency wanted the experiment to be "the 'definitive' scientific study, one that would address conflicting findings . . . and clarify issues that may have been poorly monitored in earlier studies."[23]

One important detail about USAID's support was that the agency provided funds through an open funding mechanism. They awarded a grant that was not fixed at a certain amount. This gave scientists considerable leeway to expand their study, both geographically and in terms of the scientific questions they investigated. While the initial research protocol proposed to measure only a few outcomes, such as reductions in child mortality, the research team added smaller investigations onto the main experiment. For example, the team had the money to study the impact of ITNs on the health of adolescent girls and the physical growth of primary schoolchildren, which no other research team had examined. When scientists had to expand the study population midway through the trial to achieve statistically significant results (to be discussed later in the chapter), USAID provided them with another $1 million. While USAID did not dictate the design of the experiment, the agency and its funding did shape the knowledge that scientists could produce about ITNs in Siaya.

One of the primary ways in which CDC scientists sought to produce generalizable biomedical knowledge about ITNs was to test the intervention in a community randomized controlled field trial. In 1992 one of the CDC's new field entomologists, Bill Hawley, wrote up a protocol for such an experiment, seeking to ensure that it closely resembled designs for the other TDR-sponsored bed net trials in Africa.[24] He initially designed the protocol for Mangochi in southern Malawi, where he was stationed, though these plans fell through due to personnel issues.[25] A few years later, the CDC moved the trial to Siaya, which highlights the extreme transportability of this experimental framework. Hawley revised the research protocol, again trying to align it with the procedures of the other randomized controlled trials. For Hawley and others at the CDC, the ability to compare results with other experiments in a reproducible way was key to making a global public good.

A trial measuring the efficacy of ITNs in Mangochi, or Siaya, was supposed to fill an important gap in knowledge about the intervention in regions of intense perennial transmission. Siaya residents typically experienced one hundred to three hundred infective bites each year. Scientists worried that even if ITNs reduced malaria infection among children under these conditions, it would not be enough to reduce mortality.[26] Findings from other trials, in fact, showed that the efficacy of ITNs decreased as malaria transmission pressure (the number of infectious bites per year) increased. Bernard Nahlen, who served as the director of the CDC field station in Kisian at the time, remembered that, for this reason, CDC staff did not jump at the chance to conduct the experiment. Given that the trial would be expansive, long, and costly, they wanted to ensure that they would not "spend a large part of [their] lives doing a negative study."[27]

Furthermore, in 1995 scientists working on the Kenyan coast argued that aggressively reducing malaria transmission in intense transmission areas might simply shift the age profile of the disease. For example, young children who were spared bouts of severe malaria and anemia by using ITNs might die from cerebral malaria at a slightly older age.[28] This possibility seriously concerned scientists and health officials, especially given malaria's resurgence following the cessation of eradication activities in the 1970s.[29] Some scientists worried that introducing large numbers of ITNs in Siaya might actually be harmful and delay children's acquisition of malaria immunity.[30] Such anxieties, however, did not outweigh accumulating evidence from other randomized controlled trials that the intervention reduced child mortality in Africa, even if it did so to varying degrees under different levels of transmission. These worries also did not outweigh concerns about the continent's growing malaria crisis, exacerbated by chloroquine resistance, HIV/AIDS, and the economic pressures of structural adjustment. With few other options for reducing the malaria burden in Africa, then, KEMRI-CDC moved forward with the trial, beginning research activities in 1996.

Setting up and conducting this large-scale community trial required substantially more work and planning than KEMRI-CDC's previous experiments with insecticide-treated materials. Competition from other international research organizations, such as the US Army Medical Research Unit-Kenya (part of the Walter Reed Army Institute of Research), for potential research participants in Siaya complicated this process.[31] As initially conceived, the study enrolled a population of about 55,000—most of Asembo's residents— for a two-year experiment. Scientists investigated many different epidemiological, clinical, entomological, and social scientific outcomes for this trial, including the effects of ITNs on child mortality, malaria immunity, malaria morbidity, mosquito populations, and the intervention's cost-effectiveness. Assessing any one outcome required a coordinated effort from people with different skill sets and expertise together with cooperation from trial participants. Due to their proficiency in conducting epidemiological studies, CDC staff designed the randomized controlled trial, defined its outcomes, and chose methods for measuring these outcomes. Actually applying this kind of transportable scientific expertise in Siaya, however, required CDC scientists to learn from and rely heavily on Kenyan research staff.

Making Local Claims in Siaya

For KEMRI and CDC scientists, making claims about the universality of insecticide-treated nets entailed first making local and specific claims about the efficacy of the intervention in Siaya. Scientists had to transform the area into a representative experimental site to bolster the applicability of their findings outside western Kenya. To do this, however, they had to continually tailor their research practices to circumstances there. Using what the historian Lyn Schumaker calls a "field science perspective," this section elucidates the various types of work scientists and their partners did to conduct a randomized controlled trial in Siaya and to define ITNs as universally applicable biomedical technologies.[32] This practice of global health science did not merely involve highly specialized mobile bodies of knowledge; it also included locally situated expertise, such as the ability to navigate social and political relationships in the region, which were more the purview of resident health workers than of the scientists overseeing the experiment.

Coordinating experts and expertise

This trial drew together people with a wide range of backgrounds, experience, and familiarity with Siaya. Most of the scientists who worked on the trial came to western Kenya during the 1990s—a transition moment in malaria research when there was a greater focus on the disease's clinical manifestation, as opposed to its environmental context. This was also a period during which it became clear that antimalarial drugs could not contain rising malaria rates on the continent, thus spurring research on prevention measures suitable for rural areas.[33] Hawley, his fellow entomologist John Vulule, and the immunologist Simon Kariuki had been with KEMRI-CDC since the days of the Asembo Bay Cohort Study. Vulule had, in fact, worked on some of the partnership's early bed net research in Uriri, earning his doctorate on a prescient study of mosquito resistance to pyrethroids. Bernard

Nahlen, an infectious disease specialist with the CDC, had arrived as director of the field station during the early stages of the cohort study as well. The clinical epidemiologist Feiko ter Kuile and his wife, the epidemiologist Penny Phillips-Howard, came in 1995 specifically for the ITN trial after working on malaria research elsewhere in the tropics. Phillips-Howard, one among the minority of female scientists who worked on bed net trials during this period, was initially tasked with running the social science component until it became clear that her background made her better suited to coordinating day-to-day field operations. She soon joined Hawley as a co–principal investigator, and the social scientist Jane Alaii, who was originally from Siaya, took her place.[34] Others, including the entomologists Evan Mathenge and John Gimnig and the epidemiologist S. Patrick Kachur, joined the trial during the early stages of their careers, honing their scientific skills while trying to navigate the idiosyncrasies of bed net research in rural western Kenya.[35]

The KEMRI-CDC scientists could not conduct this trial in Siaya without consulting the Kenyan government. The team hired a public health officer, Amos Odhacha from the Kenyan Ministry of Health, to be a liaison between KEMRI-CDC and the ministry and between district health teams and other research organizations working in the area. Originally a specialist in environmental health science, Odhacha had been working with the ministry for many years when he joined the staff of a primary health care project in western Kenya in the early 1990s.[36] He collaborated with the CDC on that project, leveraging this connection to get a position on the ITN trial. While Odhacha helped run insecticide treatment activities and other fieldwork during the experiment, he played an equally important role in communicating with different stakeholders to facilitate KEMRI-CDC's operations in the region. This effort to produce global health knowledge depended heavily on people like Odhacha who functioned within national organizations and networks—a persistent theme in Kenya's history with global health research.[37]

The number of professional scientists who worked on the trial paled in comparison to the hundreds of fieldworkers, drivers, data managers, and other Kenyan staff hired for the endeavor. KEMRI-CDC brought on former research staff from the Asembo Bay Cohort Project, including Michael Onyango as the field coordinator and George Okoth as a sector supervisor. They and a number of their colleagues lived in Siaya and had gained experience collecting data, mosquitoes, and other specimens around Asembo Bay on the earlier study.[38] KEMRI-CDC hired additional people from Asembo based on interviews and recommendations from Onyango and other personnel.[39] Although at the time the CDC researchers thought they were hiring fieldworkers through a mostly independent evaluation process, it became clear that Asembo residents often self-selected people, including village chiefs and those already in managerial positions, to interview for the work.[40] As Kachur recalled, communities frequently put forward their best and brightest for these positions to keep them from leaving the area in search of salaried jobs, which were few and far between in Siaya.[41]

Since these positions carried a certain degree of status and authority, scientists had to negotiate the hiring process carefully. They did not want to hire too many community leaders affiliated with the Kenya African National Union—Kenya's ruling party of the time—as most of those living in Asembo supported the opposition National Development Party, led by the Luo politician, Raila Odinga.[42] Hiring field staff was a balancing act. Project leaders had to recruit trusted and experienced people from the study area to ensure residents' cooperation, while at the same time showing themselves to be impartial. Some residents had lingering suspicions that selections were being made unfairly from within certain social and political networks. Even so, the fact that communities could recommend certain of their members for field staff positions facilitated the conduct of ITN research in the area.

While supervisors, coordinators, and other managers working in the field were mostly men—initially about 90%—many of those who gathered data from households and addressed day-to-day issues for study participants were women. The research team hired women for these tasks because they wanted people who could talk easily with families, particularly mothers, about sensitive issues like a child's death. They specifically sought out midwives, preferring those who had worked in community health care or research projects in the past. A former *nyamrerwa* I spoke with said she had learned midwifery at the Saradidi Community Health Centre and worked as a midwife before joining the trial.[43] Not all who worked as *nyamrerwa* on the trial came with midwifery experience, however. The scientists needed hundreds to conduct the trial, so they asked village communities to select people they thought could walk door to door and "keep the community's secrets."[44] Sometimes communities selected women whom they considered trustworthy but who had no prior involvement in health work. For Siaya residents, producing biomedical knowledge about ITNs was not a dispassionate or detached scientific activity, but one with considerable social meaning and consequence.

Other technical and support staff also played vital roles in the experiment, though the type of work they did does not always figure into images of global health science. In a period before the mass use of mobile phones, drivers were crucial in transporting people, objects, and data between the study site and laboratory facilities in Kisian. As with field staff, some drivers used their work on the trial to launch future work with KEMRI-CDC, which became an increasingly important employer in the region as it transformed into a hub of medical research. KEMRI-CDC also needed data managers to verify and "clean" data (e.g., removing inaccurate records) for the trial. The KEMRI administrator Benta Kamire recalled that while many people in the Kisumu area had "computer knowledge," few had those specialized data management skills.[45] Recruiting data managers from Maseno, Moi, and Kenyatta Universities, KEMRI-CDC greatly expanded the research infrastructure in Nyanza for the ITN trial.

Making the field

Besides enrolling this vast network of personnel from around the country and the globe, the KEMRI-CDC team also had to define the field. Field trials are intended to test interventions in situ, as if researchers are unobtrusive observers. Not only do researchers reorganize social relations when conducting field trials, however, creating new hierarchies separating observers from the observed; they also stabilize "the field" as a kind of laboratory, as a place where they can produce knowledge considered valid outside a specific local context.[46] For KEMRI and CDC scientists, this involved transforming Siaya's environment and population into measurable data points. In 1995, before the team distributed nets for the experiment, Hawley and the CDC statistician Allen Hightower walked around and mapped every household and geographic feature in the study area (originally just Asembo).[47] The team also took a census of everyone in the area, expanding what they had done for the Asembo Bay Cohort Project. This work aimed to establish the field's spatial and physical relations, helping researchers track things like study participants, their bed nets, data forms, and fieldworkers' cash salaries. While this mapping exercise by no means fixed Asembo residents in place—and may have stirred residents' suspicions of theft, exploitation, or other harm—it helped stabilize experimental conditions.[48]

Part of this mapping work entailed defining and bounding villages, since the experiment used villages, not individuals, as the unit of analysis. In one way, this made sense. Scientists now presumed that the insecticide on bed nets affected the distribution of mosquitoes across areas larger than an individual household. Simply tracking individuals would not account for this community-wide or "mass" effect. At the same time, defining "villages" as units of analysis and in terms of geographic space is problematic for testing an intervention such as ITNs. For one thing, villages in Siaya could be difficult to define as their boundaries tended to be fluid. Defining clear boundaries created artificial social units that did not account for people's day-to-day patterns of movement and the ways in which they encountered mosquitoes and mosquito breeding sites. Asembo residents were highly mobile, even in the evening and early morning hours when *Anopheles* mosquitoes typically feed. During funerals—an almost weekly occurrence in Siaya during the concurrent AIDS epidemic—friends and family would stay with grieving families, sometimes sleeping outside for night vigils.[49] Some children left home very early in the morning to go to school in other villages. Men from Siaya have long traveled to Kisumu and Bondo town for short-term employment. During the trial, some brought their bed nets with them while traveling.[50] The dynamic social world of Siaya and Nyanza Province burst open the containers that clinical epidemiology provided for it (albeit not in a way that compromised the experiment's internal validity).[51]

The research team also tried to define the field by collecting the demographic data of the study population, including their ethnic background, gender, and age group. They interviewed residents about sleeping behaviors and designed surveys to measure changes in mothers' perceptions of malaria and bed nets during the trial.[52] Scientists working on previous ITN trials had collected this same information to understand factors that affected people's uptake or rejection of the intervention. In fact, applied social scientific research became a key part of these trials, as research teams sought to ensure participants' cooperation and prepared to implement ITN programs after the experiments ended. Phillips-Howard initially assumed that collecting these data would simply be a matter of "tick[ing] the boxes," gathering enough surface-level data to fulfill protocol requirements.[53] It quickly became apparent to her and the rest of the team that they needed a much more detailed understanding of residents' perceptions and behaviors to carry out their clinical and epidemiological research.

Translating research in Siaya

Scientists recognized the need to tailor research plans to local conditions early on, particularly in trying to convince Siaya's residents to participate in the experiment. This process was complicated by the fact that residents held preconceived notions of researchers' motivations and what "research" would entail, as historians and anthropologists have examined elsewhere.[54] Since village chiefs wielded significant authority as gatekeepers, scientists approached them at the beginning of the trial to ensure their cooperation and blessing. According to Onyango, some chiefs worked for the CDC on the project, making them more than willing to allow the experiment. Chiefs convened *barazas* to tell residents about the trial and hear their concerns.[55] Members of the research team also held special meetings at schools, market centers, and other central locations to explain the study to people. Here, they relied heavily on Odhacha, Onyango, Okoth, and other Dholuo-speaking staff to translate project goals and activities into the local language.

The process of translating KEMRI-CDC's ITN experiment for the study population required much more than translating from English to Dholuo. When the researchers went to obtain consent from trial participants, for instance, they had to tailor their explanations of what the experiment entailed. Rather than claim that KEMRI-CDC wanted to test children's blood for signs of anemia, the consent form explained that the investigators were testing for "lack of blood."[56] Members of the research team also framed the project as an endeavor to intervene in public health locally rather than to produce global health knowledge. "As you know," the first line of the form begins, "your village is taking part in the CDC/KEMRI bednet study which aims to improve the health of young children and pregnant women in Asembo."[57] The consent form also promised participants free treatment or hospital referral for sick children. This is likely the reason that one elderly woman in Asembo could not recall participating in bed net research but did remember "signing up for hospital" with KEMRI-CDC.[58] Thinking back, Phillips-Howard guessed that many people did not fully understand the purpose of the trial even though a representative from every participating household signed the consent form. This may have been more the case for women and children, since men often signed consent forms for the household in the heavily patriarchal society.[59] *Nyamrerwa* had to go back to explain or clarify project goals to residents, especially other women, as the trial pushed ahead.

Persuading residents to join the study was no simple task. Many of those who refused to participate lived in the Asembo Bay Cohort Project area, where KEMRI-CDC had already been taking children's blood for a few years as part of that earlier project. Many found this practice threatening, especially because people understood blood as a measure of life and vitality associated with kinship, ancestral ties, land, and productivity.[60] Some also connected blood handling to witchcraft or believed that researchers were using the blood to make medicines to sell on the US and European markets.[61] These rumors, which were by no means unique to Siaya, fitted the region's longer history with colonial extraction and exploitation and persistent suspicions of the Kenyan government.[62]

KEMRI-CDC scientists sought to alleviate these fears by bringing chiefs and community advisory boards into the laboratories in Kisian so they could observe what the scientists were doing with the blood. These mediators would then report their observations back to residents.[63] The consent form also allowed participants to restrict certain types of testing on their children's blood or long-term blood storage for future testing. This was especially important because residents feared that scientists would test blood for HIV, a positive test for which signaled a physical and social death sentence. Truly tailored to local circumstances, KEMRI-CDC's consent form told residents who wanted to restrict certain testing to tell Onyango, who would then tell scientists.[64] The extent to which these various practices allayed residents' anxieties is uncertain, but the scientists clearly relied heavily on local authorities from Siaya to establish trust among the study participants.

Realities in the field posed challenges to scientists' research goals and designs in other ways as well. For example, KEMRI and CDC scientists remembered how difficult it was to explain randomization and why the experiment required it. While people seemed eager to receive bed nets, Kachur recalled, many were suspicious of randomization. Some thought that the Kenyan research staff primarily chose their kin to receive bed nets or put certain villages in the control group (which did not initially receive nets) because they did not like the villages' chiefs.[65] Researchers tried to make the selection process transparent by orchestrating big ceremonies during which village representatives picked the number 1 or 2 out of a hat to determine whether their village would receive bed nets or have to wait.[66] As Onyango recalled, the team chose to frame this as, "some villages are getting bed nets now, and the rest are getting bed nets later." He explained:

> What we realized was that when you tell people that the study, it will be two years. After two years you will all get nets. Some did not believe in that and say, "two years all of us will be dead." But we just, "Please two years is not a long duration." But most of them were really like "aye, aye! Two years, two years is too long. Make it six months." Some, "make it three months." . . . I just had to talk to them, "the way the study has been designed, we can only get that data if it is done two years."[67]

Randomized controlled trials may seem like highly standardized, mobile experimental techniques that can be conducted anywhere, but that image ignores the significant social work done by people such as Onyango to maintain this scientific framework.

The intervention at the center of this randomized controlled trial—ITNs—presented an additional obstacle, as most Siaya residents had never used a bed net. The majority understood bed nets as luxury items for blocking nuisance insects and associated the devices with foreigners, government employees, and the wealthy. Since most people did not connect malaria to mosquitoes—instead believing that the illness was caused by rain, cold, eating rotten fruit, or witchcraft—they also did not internalize the connection between using a bed net and preventing malaria.[68] As they distributed bed nets, then, the research staff demonstrated how people were supposed to hang the nets above sleeping spaces in their homes, including mats and sofas where children often slept. They gave out leaflets describing how to properly care for the nets.[69] Getting people to assimilate bed nets into their household furniture, however, proved difficult using these methods alone. When staff carried out a house-to-house monitoring campaign in the month before the intervention period was supposed to begin, they found that, in roughly half the homes they visited, people did not have nets hung correctly or had not even taken nets out of the package.[70] Dholuo-speaking field staff again played a critical role in communicating how and why people should use this technology, which would be essential to the experiment.

Making biomedical knowledge in Siaya

After much planning, preparation, and negotiation, KEMRI-CDC scientists finally began to collect data on whether ITNs could reduce child mortality. Again, this was easier said than done. A few months into the trial, in early 1997, Alaii and some of her CDC colleagues conducted a participatory rural appraisal—a survey that gathers the opinions of people living in rural communities, so programmers can then incorporate those opinions into projects implemented in those communities. They found that many people were still either not using the nets or not sleeping entirely underneath them every night. Persistent gaps in understanding the public health utility of this object played a role, as did residents' previous encounters with health projects, the government, and other outsiders. Some felt that ITNs were actually tools scientists would use to draw people's blood secretly while they slept. Because Nyanza had been a major site for family planning projects in the past, some thought that these nets, dosed with pungent chemicals, were tools of sterilization. They were especially wary that the government, represented by KEMRI, was trying to reduce the population of this opposition-supporting region—a fear observed in various public health campaigns across the continent over the late twentieth- and twenty-first centuries.[71] And some recipients did not think the ITNs were truly free. They worried that scientists would ask people to pay for the net if they were found using it, and if they did not have the money, scientists would take their land instead.[72]

Residents avoided nets for more obvious reasons as well. Many found it hot and uncomfortable to sleep under a net. With upward of 156 holes per square inch, nets inhibit ventilation as well as malarious mosquitoes. Some people also stopped sleeping under their nets during the hot and dry season, when noisier, more perceptible benign mosquitoes were less prevalent but the threat of malaria-carrying *Anopheles* remained. The insecticide provided its own discomfort. When people touched the insecticide on the net before it had fully dried, they would develop a rash or start to itch. Some recalled that the chemical provoked coughing fits, heightening suspicions that nets could kill their children.[73] While a majority of trial participants—according to one survey, about 70%—ultimately used the intervention as intended during the trial, many others did not due to sensory perceptions, social preconceptions, and an altogether different understanding of how the technology worked.[74] Initial efforts to educate the study participants and control the use of nets as a health-promoting tool, it seemed, did not fully address these material imaginaries and realities.

To produce biomedical knowledge, researchers had to adapt to residents' ideas and practices, often working through those that were already embedded in and familiar to communities in Siaya. To ensure that people used their nets, Alaii and other Siaya-based staff did random evening spot checks with the help of community elders. *Nyamrerwa* visited "refusal homesteads" to assuage fears about using ITNs.[75] Many people also confided in Onyango, who mediated between scientists and participants: "I . . . t[old] them that, 'I cannot bring something bad to you because I will be here forever,'" he recalled. "'If there is anything wrong, you may blame me forever.'"[76] Such promises of longevity, which stood in contrast to the unpredictable and time-limited nature of research projects, helped maintain residents' participation and trust in the project.

Along those lines, early adopters among study participants were also important to building trust in the intervention. Women who used ITNs continued to bear children. Young children of families using the nets did not get sick with fever as often as before. Of course, not all children who slept in households with ITNs survived, and in those cases the families continued to think nets were dangerous.[77] Nevertheless, those who observed that net-using neighbors were okay—especially at a time when many young children in Asembo died from malaria and febrile illness—were more likely to use them too.

Researchers did not rely simply on personal conversations to address this issue of people not using their nets. Alaii and Phillips-Howard also altered their communication and education strategies in ways they felt were better suited to Siaya. For example, they had staff talk with participants about the proper use of nets during meetings of church and women's groups since more people attended these than chiefs' *barazas*. Unlike some outreach activities used in the lead-up to the trial, such as football matches where scientists explained the experiment to the players, these meetings more specifically targeted women, who were much more vulnerable to malaria while pregnant and were typically the primary caretakers of young children.[78] The research team also organized drawing contests in schools where children drew pictures about proper bed net use and treatment with insecticide. They staged theater shows about ITNs and held ceremonies where *nyamrerwa* sang songs about the trial.[79] These "community"-oriented education activities underscore that getting people to use this new technology as a malaria control tool required substantial engagement with intended users. Merely providing access was insufficient.

Scientists also considered giving gifts to ensure people's participation. Onyango and the lead investigators discussed the possibility of offering incentives to mothers who allowed blood to be drawn from their placenta upon giving birth or answered questions about their child's death.[80] The fact that many in the region believed it was important to either bury the placenta near their house or dispose of it properly to ensure the safety, growth, and belonging of a newborn made it all the more important to broach these research practices carefully.[81] Since residents frequently asked the researchers for coffins, which were expensive, Phillips-Howard recalled, the team initially considered giving these as incentives to mothers whose child had died. They ultimately decided against this because mothers "might connect the death, as if it is now the bed net project which is causing deaths and we [project staff] are aware."[82] They decided instead to offer small incentives to mothers at birth to provide placental blood within six hours of delivery "because," Onyango explained, "this is like welcoming" the child. "You have to motivate this family that when they give birth, they can keep that placenta."[83] KEMRI-CDC also paid *nyamrerwa* per delivery, encouraging them to attend births and help collect information from mothers.

Asembo residents' mobility posed further difficulties in running this experiment. During funerals, many family members from outside Asembo would come to stay in households involved in the trial. Hosts would often let visitors use their nets, which may have caused the data to suggest lower ITN efficacy.[84] Sometimes visitors would take the nets with them when they left the area. Onyango remembered going all the way to Kisumu to retrieve a net from the trial, a trip that took at least a couple of hours to complete.[85] Mobility proved a considerable thorn in the side of scientists throughout the experiment, as much as they tried to control it.

The insecticide component of the intervention presented unanticipated challenges as well. According to the research protocol, scientists and other field staff had to re-treat the bed nets with insecticide every six months to maintain their potency. Staff told participants to bring their nets to a central location where they would then dip the nets in permethrin. Scientists described this to me as a drill, an activity that required an army working for one month twice a year. For some, the treatment process was simply a "nightmare."[86] As with many other aspects of the trial, the encroachment of research protocols into private and intimate spheres of residents' lives created problems. Some considered nets as part of their private bedding—materials associated with reproduction, fertility, and bodily contact—and thus refused to show their bed nets in public.[87] While not unique among African communities, their refusal surprised researchers like Odhacha, who told me, "I'm a

Luo, but some things I didn't know."[88] Early surveys conducted to understand the compatibility of participants' sleeping habits with the experiment's intervention did not interrogate these deeper meanings and social norms regarding bed nets. ITNs may appear to be simple, obvious public health tools, but this bed net trial and others from the continent highlighted that this was not always the case.

Dipping nets in insecticide was also difficult because many participants had concerns about dipping their nets in a communal washbasin. Some men did not want to have their nets dipped in the same insecticide solution that was just used to treat the net of a menstruating girl, possibly because of menstruation's associations with sexuality and cultural ideas about the risks of improper mixing of bodies and bodily substances.[89] Family hierarchy also mattered as some men, Vulule recalled, wanted their net dipped before that of their daughter-in-law.[90] People asked to have nets treated at their homes so they could more easily control the process. Since this would be incredibly time consuming and logistically challenging, the research team instead had to learn to negotiate village, homestead, and household relationships in the communal dipping process.[91] This kind of social labor was critical to ensuring that scientists could measure the effects of this public health intervention, which they had introduced into an existing world of materials dense with social and cultural meaning.

And even as prepared and well-funded as KEMRI-CDC was, it found that getting insecticide to the study site could be quite precarious. In August 1998 the US Embassy in Nairobi was bombed. Since the embassy had been the waypoint for all incoming insecticide for the study, the attack caused a nine- to twelve-month delay in getting this crucial ingredient to Siaya for the trial.[92] Like people's refusal to dip their nets in insecticide, this delay threatened to change the identity of the intervention being tested. Scientists folded this incident into their research findings, using the experience to demonstrate that the efficacy of ITNs declined markedly if not treated after six months.[93] Circumstances in Siaya and Kenya more broadly shaped the knowledge that scientists produced about this object, as well as the character of the technology they tested at any given moment.

Scientists' clinical and epidemiological investigations impinged on many participants' feelings of comfort and safety because this research required the extraction of life-sustaining bodily fluids and intrusions into domestic life, reproduction, and social rituals. While not nearly as intrusive, their investigation of the effects of ITNs on mosquitoes also raised questions from residents. Entomologists had to hang Columbian curtains (nets that hang off eaves) around people's houses in the evenings to collect mosquitoes flying out, a process that many participants found entertaining and struggled to understand. "Some were at times amused," Vulule recalled. "Why are we chasing mosquitoes? Because whereas they appreciate the fact that mosquitoes might cause malaria, just to have our vehicles driving around chasing mosquitoes . . . at times they couldn't fathom why we had so much interest."[94] Mathenge, who came from Nairobi to work on the trial, similarly remembered that people would ask him why he "would come all this way just to chase mosquitoes."[95] If this trial was an orchestration of people, activities, knowledge, and skills, it was one in which not every player knew what was going on or why. This incomplete understanding went both ways, even if it was not entirely symmetrical.

Maintaining mobility and the field

Asembo was not the only place where scientists and research staff produced knowledge about ITNs for the trial. Laboratories in Kisian also functioned as an important center of knowledge production, though it was tethered to the rural field site. The research team did cross-sectional surveys each year during the trial. Intensive data collection in the field developed into intensive work in the lab. "We did those cross-sectional surveys for about one month or six weeks," Simon Kariuki told me. He continued:

> And it involved everyday waking up around five in the morning, so that [KEMRI-CDC field researchers] will be in the field. If they have to leave Kisumu and be in the field by eight, they had to leave at five, and pass by the labs, pick the drugs, pick the ice packs for samples, and whatever supplies they needed to go to the field. . . . And then if [the children surveyed] have fever, then the slides will be brought here and given priority and had to be read first so that the next day [researchers] can take the drugs in the field. So by the time they finish all that, back in the lab it's about nine P.M. at night. And then you have to process those samples, and so on, until one A.M. Sometimes people in the lab would leave at one A.M. And the next day by five, six A.M. they needed to be back in the lab.[96]

Indeed, scientists and their staff did not simply conduct the trial in Siaya. Rather, this field experiment unfolded through the transcontinental circulation of people, objects, knowledge, and capital. The last leg of this movement from Kisian to Siaya could sometimes be the most difficult and precarious to complete.[97] *Nyamrerwa* and field staff collected data for thousands of people on standardized paper forms, which drivers transported between Siaya and Kisian in land cruisers on a regular basis. If someone in Kisian wanted to follow up with a participant about their response on the paper forms, he or she had to physically go to Asembo and find that person. Scientists who wanted to provide people with the results of their blood test had to supply drivers with tiny scraps of paper containing information on where to find them.[98] Benta Kamire recalled that much of her work as an administrator at the time entailed maintaining the circulation of paper, cash salaries for field staff, and other materials to ensure the experiment's success.[99]

This experiment required a lot of work and coordination, but that is only the half of it. Much of what has been described so far has been about activities in Asembo. Based on census data from the early 1990s, CDC scientists thought a trial with around 55,000–60,000 participants in Asembo would be enough to show a 20% reduction in child mortality due to ITN use. Census data from 1996—the year scientists planned to distribute nets—showed, however, that child mortality in Asembo was lower than researchers expected. Low child mortality rates meant it would be more difficult to show that ITN use was the cause of any increase in child survival. High HIV-related mortality in the study area also meant it would be especially difficult to demonstrate that a malaria control tool could save lives.[100] Frantically recalculating how many people they would need to maintain the study's statistical power (and minimize the probability that the experiment would fail to detect a true effect), Allen Hightower and Feiko ter Kuile reported that the team needed to include about 70,000 more people.[101] This meant they had to do everything over again in the location of Gem, to the north, all while continuing to collect and analyze data from Asembo.

The research infrastructure set up by KEMRI-CDC in Gem was much sparser than that in Asembo and was geared mainly toward measuring reductions in child mortality, the primary outcome of interest. As a result, the Gem study area was more difficult to oversee. CDC scientists acknowledged that, in the end, it was hard to assess ITN use in Gem in detail. According to ter Kuile, things that slipped under their radar, such as when people siphoned off insecticide to use for agricultural purposes, probably diluted results.[102] The compound nature of this technology, comprising both insecticide and bed nets, made it a much more challenging intervention to control and eval-uate compared to a drug or vaccine.

Taking a field science perspective, this account of KEMRI-CDC's ITN trial reveals a complex performance of global health science. Conducting the ex-periment required many people using different types of skills and expertise. Although the CDC scientists defined what they wanted and needed to have done to make knowledge usable for other scientists, policy makers, and do-nor agencies around the world, they could not have made local and specific claims about ITNs in Siaya on their own. Communicating, socializing, trav-eling, and being present were critical to the production of biomedical knowl-edge about this object. Only by looking at these practices and the many people involved in this work, is it possible to understand the labor required to make ITNs function as biomedical technologies in a place where most people did not understand them as such.

Disseminating Results

The intervention period for the trial wrapped up in 2000, once the researchers completed the second year of data collection for Gem. While the scientists produced many findings from this massive study, including that the use of insecticide-treated nets did not seem to compromise children's ma-laria immunity, they produced two important findings in particular. First, statistical results showed a 20% reduction in all-cause child mortality among children under five years old and a 26% reduction among children under one year old specifically.[103] Infants in Siaya benefited the most from sleeping under ITNs, since the device reduced the number of infectious bites they received and, in turn, their risk for severe anemia. Scientists converted these statistics into numbers of "lives saved," calculating 10 lives saved per 1,000 child years for children under the age of five and 35 lives saved per 1,000 child years for those under the age of one.[104] The techniques of clinical epide-miology had effectively distilled out the biomedical effects of ITNs, leav-ing behind the process of achieving those effects as negligible residue.

Second, entomologists' data showed that ITNs had a "community-wide effect," sometimes called a "mass effect" or "herd effect." Hawley and his col-leagues did a spatial analysis of epidemiological data to show that children in compounds within 300 meters of households using ITNs experienced sim-ilar reductions in disease indicators compared to those of children using those nets.[105] Some entomologists noted a mass effect in earlier studies, but not all malaria researchers agreed on this point. Scientists also did not know how strong the mass effect was, assuming it existed.[106] Accounting for this mass effect and the additional lives a single net could save, health economists reduced the estimated cost of saving lives with ITN use.[107] Mobilizing quantitative evidence that ITNs had a community-wide effect, CDC scientists bolstered the argument that donors should provide the intervention for free to pregnant women and children under the age of five.[108] Statistical results reduced ITNs to their ability to save lives, though, of course, the technology's ability to do so depended on whether most people regularly slept under and treated their bed nets—an endeavor that scientists struggled to achieve even in ideal, controlled experimental conditions.

The research team disseminated these results to various stakeholders, including study participants, fieldworkers, Kenyan health officials, and members of the international health community. In communicating with international stakeholders in particular, they generalized claims they had made about the efficacy of ITNs in Siaya, defining ITNs as universally applicable and substantiating calls to distribute the intervention in all malaria-affected areas of Africa. They held ceremonies in Kisumu and Nairobi to report their results for the Ministry of Health and major donors. Filled with music and speeches, these ceremonies functioned as displays of international support for malaria control in Kenya. Scientists also brought fieldworkers into the Kisian field station to report the results, where they received certificates of accomplishment. Not merely for show, these paper tokens have come to function as claims that community health workers make to status and experience to secure work on other research projects.[109]

As promised, KEMRI-CDC gave out bed nets to members of the control group and shared what they had found with Siaya's residents. It was "exciting information to the community," Odhacha told me, that malaria, not witchcraft, was the culprit in so many child deaths in the area, and now they could use bed nets to protect themselves.[110] Although, it is difficult to recapture residents' genuine attitudes about bed nets from nearly twenty years ago, many people I spoke with in 2015 said that they appreciated bed nets because now they and their family members did not get sick with malaria as often: "You could go to the hospital for other things," one woman told me, "but not for malaria."[111]

Beyond Kenya, scientists presented findings to officials at the World Health Organization (WHO), at academic conferences, and in journals. They also disseminated trial results through the American media and popular science publications—a sign that ITNs had truly made it onto the global health stage. "The study also shows," one article read, "that a remarkably low-tech and relatively cheap intervention can have more impact than many snazzy scientific advances."[112] Citing findings from the trial showing that ITNs had a "herd effect," the author reinforced claims from scientists that the devices were cost-effective, global public goods.[113] Meanwhile, the construction of ITNs as "remarkably low-tech" (in contrast to a vaccine or other types of "snazzy scientific advances") in public and fundraising arenas further downplayed the need to consider local contexts of use. What was anything but simple for KEMRI-CDC scientists carrying out a highly controlled experiment became a simple, self-evident global health technology.

It is important to note, though, that policy makers at the WHO included ITNs in their new Roll Back Malaria campaign before KEMRI and CDC scientists published results from the Siaya trial. "Although we were sure that this was the most important study that was being done, was going to answer the question about whether or not the nets worked in a very high transmission area," Kachur remembered, "I knew the rest of the world wasn't sitting around on their hands waiting for those results. They were moving forward. But the direction that they were moving forward was on a rather smallish scale and focused a lot on developing ways to make it possible for people to afford to buy a bed net, or to afford to buy the insecticide retreatment once they had it."[114] The trial answered many open questions about the efficacy of ITNs, but the results strengthened support for, rather than significantly change the direction of global malaria control. "At the international level," Phillips-Howard recalled, "it was the lobbying and the demanding for, 'look at all these deaths. They can be prevented. We need more money. This isn't going to happen unless bed nets get out there. You must treat this as a social vaccine.' You know, 'we've been able to dot the i's and cross the t's with this study, and it needs to move forward as a public good.'"[115] As many CDC scientists told me, the fact that scientists could now provide statistics showing that ITNs worked anywhere was important for stimulating enthusiasm about nets among donors. ITNs and the statistically articulated, biomedical claims now firmly attached to or embedded in the technology were construed and disseminated as global public goods.

Scientists compiled and published results in a single supplement for the *American Journal of Tropical Medicine and Hygiene* in 2003. They did not do so simply to create a storehouse of biomedical knowledge about ITNs; they also wanted the journal supplement to be a policy and public health teaching tool. The supplement included articles on the feasibility of using demographic surveillance systems instead of statistics from government health facilities to track the health of rural populations—findings that justified distributing ITNs to control malaria without improving health facilities, for which there were few resources.[116] Phillips-Howard and her coauthors wrote extensive descriptions relating how KEMRI-CDC set up and conducted the trial so other researchers could use the bed net experiment as a model for large randomized controlled field trials in impoverished, rural settings.[117] Like scientific results from the trial and ITNs, this journal supplement was a product designed for global consumption.

Just as local contexts influence global health knowledge, so too does global health science affect the places where it is conducted. KEMRI-CDC's ITN trial had a major impact on Siaya and the VBCRC as places for medical research. Beginning with the Asembo Bay Cohort Project, KEMRI and CDC scientists transformed areas of Siaya into health and demographic surveillance sites where researchers could monitor hundreds of households through networks of local health workers. They expanded surveillance activities significantly during the ITN trial to cover most of Asembo and Gem. Teams working on later medical research projects or tracking bed net coverage in Siaya used the same surveillance infrastructure to collect data from thousands of rural households. USAID and other donors started to give substantial amounts of funding to the center because it had the capacity to collect data from large populations, allocating a lot of money for HIV/AIDS research. In part because the center started getting so much financial support to study HIV/AIDS, which is not vector borne, leadership changed the name of the institution to the KEMRI Centre for Global Health Research around 2004.[118] Through KEMRI-CDC's ITN trial, the center, along with Siaya, had become a central hub for global health science in Africa—including one of the first population-level trials of a malaria vaccine in 2009.

ITNs did not begin their life as a biomedical technology. Neither scientists nor bed net users understood these as objects that reduced malaria disease or mortality, at least not initially. For a long time, malaria experts believed that this tool might not have the same health effects everywhere. Fears that ITNs might not work in areas of intense malaria transmission, in fact, led scientists from the CDC and KEMRI to conduct a major randomized controlled trial of the intervention in Siaya in the mid-1990s. In the process of conducting this experiment, they cemented the identity of ITNs as universally applicable biomedical tools.

This moment in ITNs' trajectory as scientific objects cannot be reduced simply to a case where scientists ignored the importance of local circumstances to their work. KEMRI and CDC scientists were very aware of how conditions on the ground affected the way they produced knowledge about nets. They learned through their experience on the trial that the social and cultural world of Siaya informed scientific results, and could even alter them. Moreover, they learned that fieldworkers who had lived and worked in the study sites were instrumental to the production of biomedical knowledge about this health intervention.

However, the process of scaling up, or generalizing, knowledge from this specific experiment to generate global health knowledge transformed Siaya into a backdrop for knowledge production rather than an integral part of it. In disseminating the experiment's findings, particularly through statistical data, scientists helped reify ITNs as tools that could save lives no matter where they traveled. As subsequent chapters explore in greater detail, policy makers and donors took up and circulated this vision of ITNs as a "remarkably low-tech" and cost-effective means of saving lives, leaving Siaya out of the picture completely. The ways in which people used this technology and assimilated it into their daily lives became detached from the function of the technology itself. Looking at the life of ITNs as scientific objects over the 1980s and 1990s not only showcases Africans' important roles in the development of global health science and interventions; it also illustrates how the development of global health science, and its emphasis on randomized controlled trials and biomedical knowledge, obscured the impact of local contingencies on malaria control.

3

The Technology of Neoliberal Policy

Taking Insecticide-Treated Nets to Market

In April 2000 multitudes of political and business leaders descended on Abuja, Nigeria, for the first Summit to Roll Back Malaria in Africa. The Nigerian president, Olusegun Obasanjo, members of Nigeria's Ministry of Health, and other state officials welcomed visitors from across the continent and the globe. Though heterogeneous in their professional backgrounds, all these visitors gathered to promote and publicize malaria control in Africa, which until then had been a marginal cause on the world health agenda. Nigerian children sang and danced, while photographers from international media outlets snapped pictures. In the week leading up to the summit meeting, the Nigerian First Lady, Stella Obasanjo, unveiled what appeared to be a giant mesh circus tent on the parade grounds of Eagle Square. More than 200 Nigerian children crowded under the structure—a world record-breaking bed net—to give onlookers a sense of how many African children died from malaria every two and a half hours and thus the number of lives insecticide-treated nets could save. This "somewhat bizarre publicity stunt with a serious message" kicked off a milestone conference, where high-ranking officials, including the director-general of the World Health Organization (WHO), Gro Harlem Brundtland, spoke passionately to delegates about a new global effort to roll back malaria (and "Roll in Development"): "We now have an extraordinary window of opportunity. We have governments, international organisations, NGOs [nongovernmental organizations] and the private sector ready to work together to achieve agreed health goals and so contribute to prosperity."[1] ITNs, as Brundtland, Obasanjo, and their fellow attendees indicated, would play a starring role in this public-private endeavor.

Chapters 1 and 2 described the long, contingent process by which ITNs became understood as evidence-based biomedical technologies. In short, scientists conducted randomized controlled trials demonstrating that this tool could save children's lives and economists calculated its cost-effectiveness—metrics that international health donors increasingly used to evaluate interventions and rationalize their investments during the 1980s and 1990s.[2] The identity of ITNs as scientifically validated, lifesaving objects alone, however, does not explain the technology's rise to prominence at the turn of the twenty-first century. ITNs acquired an additional persona, established partly through field experiments and pilot projects, that proved equally important to their adoption as a cornerstone of Roll Back Malaria policy. As cheap commodities, which fit easily into decentralized, market-based models of public health, ITNs served as tools for advancing and enacting neoliberal health reforms in Africa during structural adjustment. This political function appealed to leaders of influential donor agencies, which eventually joined Brundtland and the WHO in promoting economic development on the continent under the banner of malaria control.

To understand this other aspect of the emergence of ITNs as a major global health intervention, we must go back in time to the early 1980s, when many of the political and economic shifts that came to define twenty-first century global health were set in motion.[3] During this period, African governments began divesting and reforming their health sectors according to the pro-market, antistate tenets of structural adjustment, in order to access badly needed loans, debt relief, and resources from the World Bank and other development agencies. They did so as malaria rates spiked across the continent, creating a crisis that was hastened by increasing economic instability. WHO officials sought financial support from these same development agencies, which had begun to supersede the WHO in financing international health activities.[4] Both national and international health officials were now trying to find inexpensive malaria control strategies suitable for decentralized, privatized health systems to secure funding. ITNs not only fulfilled this need but also, as a prevention measure, promised to save money on costly curative services. They became concrete, tangible means of making public health in Africa a market-based activity that was capable of permeating the poorest communities of impending citizen-consumers and unlocking the coffers of global health's rising patrons. This, and not simply scientific evidence, informed the intervention's inclusion and preeminence in Roll Back Malaria policy.

In calling ITNs a technology of policy, I want to stress that the intervention did not merely reflect donors' political and economic interests. It also served as a means of implementing neoliberal health reforms, even if those reforms did not occur entirely as imagined. Other work on the history of development in Africa has similarly shown how a variety of technologies helped enact social, political, and economic change. Colonial officials remade roads in Tanganyika to control the mobility of African populations, whom they considered vectors of physical and social disease.[5] Mozambique's Frelimo government reconceptualized the Portuguese-controlled Cahora Bassa dam as a "symbol of liberation and instrument of growth," which authorities felt could help electrify the countryside and consolidate power behind the new socialist state.[6] Although ITNs may not be as obvious a technology of development as dams or transportation infrastructure, we can subject them to the same analysis to understand how health policy makers envisioned transforming public health governance in Africa at a local and material level. By doing so here, this chapter sheds new light on the ways that structural adjustment policies were implemented on the continent, particularly in the domain of public health.

Tracking the adoption of a specific technology in health policy also provides the opportunity to elucidate the dialectical relationship between national and international policy-making efforts, as well as between idealized policies and on-the-ground implementation. As the case of malaria control policy in Kenya bears out, state health officials did not always wait for international leaders to embrace ITNs before recommending that their citizens take up this tool. Even then, target users did not always adopt ITNs as policy makers envisioned.[7] Their experiences in turn informed international discussions about how best to distribute ITNs on the continent, even if influential donor agencies had a substantial say in crafting malaria control strategies.[8] Illuminating these interactions between international, national, and subnational levels of malaria control policy making highlights another avenue through which Africans and African settings shaped global health.

Reviving Malaria Control in an Age of Scarcity

Some of the same political and economic factors informing scientists' investigations of insecticide-treated nets during the 1980s also shaped the development of malaria control policies in the post-eradication period. Prevailing conditions of resource scarcity and international agencies' appeal to private and nongovernmental channels to sustain health programs on a shoestring profoundly affected official recommendations for curbing malaria in Africa.

The global economic crisis that opened the 1980s coincided with a significant decline in funding and attention for malaria. Many health and development agencies considered malaria control politically unpopular due to the perceived difficulties and high costs of the endeavor in Africa. Any investment in malaria control, they felt, might not influence health outcomes enough to justify the expense or, even worse, could lead to rebounds in malaria after funding dried up. The dearth of effective tools also discouraged action. The epidemiologist Don de Savigny, who worked on bed net research in Tanzania and became heavily involved in international bed net programming, remembered this shortage well: "UNICEF [the United Nations Children's Fund] was big on vaccines, it was big on nutrition, it was big on many things. But there was zero on malaria because there was nothing they could do."[9] Malaria control activities, based largely on the dispensation of antimalarial drugs, became subsumed into nascent, under-resourced primary health care services in many African countries.

The economic crisis also affected public health spending more generally. The WHO, a traditional leader in the field of international health, struggled to maintain incoming donations, especially as wealthy donors voiced their skepticism about the organization's effectiveness. When malaria rates began to rise in Africa in the mid-1980s, the WHO had neither the material resources nor the technical capacity to address the disease. It continued to encourage countries to integrate malaria into primary health care services, for which it could also offer limited financial support. Meanwhile, the World Bank pressured African governments to reform their health sectors according to structural adjustment policies, including by cutting health care spending and privatizing and decentralizing health services. The growing malaria crisis, absorption of malaria activities into primary health care services, and push for neoliberal health reforms on the continent provided the backdrop for late twentieth-century malaria control policy.

While certainly not universal, Kenya's experience with health policy reform and malaria represents what occurred in Africa more broadly during this transition period. The country's economy suffered a severe blow during the debt crisis of the 1970s as oil prices spiked, commodity prices fluctuated, and the East African Community collapsed in 1977. The World Bank and the International Monetary Fund (IMF) floated the first of multiple structural adjustment loans to Kenya in 1980 to help the government pay back creditors—mainly wealthy countries in the global north. In return, the Kenyan government agreed to adopt trade liberalization policies and austerity measures, reorienting its economy toward rapid economic growth. In addition, the government cut spending on social services such as health care, which even before the debt crisis relied heavily on external funding.[10] As Kenya's health system buckled under the pressure of divestment, state officials prioritized efforts to find alternative financing mechanisms for health programs. Because it was "no longer possible for the government to do everything in the health sector," Kenya's minister of health called on NGOs and the private sector to take on a greater role in health financing.[11] Following World Bank recommendations, the government ended its policy of providing free care in state health facilities, implementing user fees in 1989. These and later declarations of reform placed increasing responsibility on individuals to pay for health care, even though a large portion of the population continued to live in poverty.

The World Bank also pressured the Kenyan government to transfer responsibility for organizing health care to district officials as part of larger attempts to dismantle what bank leaders saw as a massive and obstructive central bureaucracy. The government started this devolution with its District Focus for Rural Development strategy in 1983. In practice, however, district officials only gained nominal control over health services because they did not have a means of generating revenue themselves. They still relied on funds from the central government, which President Daniel arap Moi and colleagues often distributed according to political loyalties.[12] Other development agencies, such as the United States Agency for International Development (USAID), also encouraged decentralization of health services in Kenya by funneling health funding through NGOs. Despite Moi's attempt to curb the power of NGOs in the country, donors increasingly relied on these nongovernmental actors to distribute aid during the 1990s, especially as Moi's government faced international scrutiny and sanctions for human rights abuses.[13]

To cut down on hospital-based curative services in urban areas, development agency partners also called for greater investment in cost-effective preventive services in Kenya's health reforms. The expensive tertiary care that urban hospitals provided, critics argued, diverted state funds away from programs that would address the wider burden of disease in Kenya, shouldered mainly by poor, rural populations. In practice, calls for more preventive services translated into more money for "the expansion of both demand and supply of family planning services," which the World Bank and other agencies considered critical for population control and economic growth in low-income countries.[14] Malaria control initially received little attention in Kenya's health sector reforms under structural adjustment. This reflected not only the interests and strategies of development agencies from the global north but also the dearth of resources and specially trained personnel for malaria activities in rural districts.

Yet malaria was becoming difficult to ignore in Kenya and other parts of sub-Saharan Africa. Increasing poverty and the decreasing efficacy of chloroquine exacerbated malaria mortality, especially among young children. The disease even began to ravage Kenya's "economically important highlands" in 1988, after nearly thirty years of quiescence.[15] This occurred as new agricultural development projects and population pressure forced people to live closer to mosquito breeding sites. By 1989 malaria had become a leading cause of outpatient morbidity and a major burden on health facilities in the country.[16] The AIDS crisis also compromised the safety of using blood transfusions to treat severe anemia. Kenya and other African countries sorely needed malaria mitigation measures even if policy makers focused on addressing other concerns.

International neglect of the disease came into focus at the WHO Executive Board's eighty-fifth Session in 1990, when members of the board acknowledged that "it was worth the Board's while to take time to look at the malaria question just as closely as the AIDS problem."[17] At this time, the WHO Malaria Action Programme received about $3.4 million from the WHO's regular funds and $1.4 million from extrabudgetary funding for malaria control. Lamenting the lack of attention to the current disease crisis, Malawi's chief of health services, H. M. Ntaba, called on the WHO to take action. "WHO must do a great deal more to control the disease," he stated, "including efforts to secure the support of Member States that might not be highlighting the problem not because they considered it unimportant but because in many cases their programmes were 'donor-driven' in the sense that they could be implemented only if resources from donors were available. Unless WHO put the malaria problem into its proper perspective, donors would continue to shy away from it." Ntaba "therefore hope[d] that every effort would be made to mobilize additional extrabudgetary resources, since US $1.4 million was a very inadequate sum."[18] With little optimism that the WHO would increase its own budget, establishing channels to donor funding became an important component of malaria control in Africa, just as it became a significant element of Kenya's health sector reforms.

In response to these and other appeals, the chief medical officer of the UK Department of Health, Sir Donald Acheson, proposed a global conference of ministers to help "raise the profile" of malaria.[19] Although people in wealthy countries had largely forgotten about the disease, he felt that they would soon become aware of the problem as more and more tourists returned home with malaria. The WHO's deputy director-general supported the idea, arguing that "extrabudgetary resources must be sought very actively."[20] One participant added that the WHO should spend money on cultivating interest in malaria and employing a "suitable advocate" rather than hiring another epidemiologist as initially planned.[21] Discussions at the meeting indicated that the WHO's main role in malaria control would be to generate interest in malaria from potential donors.

WHO leaders held three interregional meetings ahead of the proposed global conference to discuss the main challenges to malaria control in Africa, Latin America, and Southeast Asia, respectively. In October 1991 the WHO's Regional Office for Africa (WHO AFRO) convened a meeting at its headquarters in Brazzaville, Congo. Here, attendees focused on outlining the problems faced by under-resourced areas with highly endemic malaria, along with potential action plans and "appropriate strategies and options for the control of malaria . . . that can be sustained especially under conditions of restricted national resources."[22]

Considering such constraints, the conference participants discussed the possibility of including ITNs in malaria control activities. Some noted that the efficacy of the intervention in different epidemiological settings remained uncertain.[23] Scientists had tested ITNs only on a small scale in a few African sites by this point. Development agency representatives also questioned whether African communities would purchase bed nets and insecticide, which they felt would be critical to maintaining any new malaria control efforts on the continent. "Insecticide impregnated curtains and bednets show some promise but have not been tried on a market and consumer financed basis," the deputy assistant administrator of USAID wrote to a colleague. "Will people be willing to purchase 80% of what would be needed to protect themselves from malaria using insecticide impregnated curtains?"[24] Despite such concerns, health officials still thought the tool was promising because of its "low cost and the ease with which [insecticide] impregnation can be done by members of the community"—qualities scientists had also highlighted in their experiments.[25] The intervention's political and practical advantages ultimately led the authors of the Brazzaville conference Summary Report to call on African governments to test ITNs and curtains within their national borders. The intervention was gaining traction just as malaria control was slowly reemerging on the international health agenda.

Adopting Nets and Enacting Health Reforms in Kenya's Bamako Initiative Projects

Kenya's experience with adopting insecticide-treated nets emphasizes the extent to which new political and economic realities of the period, not just scientific evidence, influenced the trajectory of the intervention. In fact, Kenyan health officials incorporated nets into national health activities by 1990, before Medical Research Council scientists published the results of their landmark mortality trial from The Gambia in 1991. They did not do so as part of a malaria-specific campaign, but rather as part of a new primary health care program, dubbed the Bamako Initiative. The "community based" cost-recovery projects at the center of Kenya's Bamako Initiative served as a means of decentralizing and privatizing health care in the country.[26] ITNs circulated as health commodities within these projects, helping enact neoliberal health reforms as much as mitigating malaria in Kenya.

Although the country's experience with adopting ITNs was unique in some ways, it ultimately built on a longer trend in international health: the distribution of cheap, individualized health interventions through decentralized channels. In their aid programs in the late 1970s, major donor agencies such as USAID, the World Bank, and the WHO embraced the concept of "appropriate technology"—roughly defined as technology suitable to the social, economic, environmental, and cultural conditions of the place in which it is applied. Different organizations characterized appropriate technologies differently. However, by the 1980s, the US government's definition of cheap, simple, off-patent technology-commodities became predominant, as agencies sought to extend health care to poor, rural areas with limited resources and state involvement.[27] The United Nations Children's Fund (UNICEF) became a chief advocate of appropriate technologies, embracing interventions such as childhood immunizations and oral rehydration therapy for childhood diarrhea. Investment in these individualized solutions drew attention away from building up broader infrastructure, such as sewage systems or rural clinics.[28] These solutions were also easy to disseminate through private sector channels and voluntary and nongovernmental organizations, allowing aid agencies to save on infrastructure costs and bypass the central state bureaucracy.

Following this trend, the WHO and UNICEF jointly introduced the Bamako Initiative in 1987 as a plan for expanding primary health care in Africa using revolving fund schemes. In these schemes, individuals paid slightly higher prices for basic health commodities—often in pharmacies, other retail outlets, or clinics—to replenish supplies and cover health worker salaries. Ideally, this would help communities maintain drug stocks and further extend health care to areas underserved by government health resources, which, given the political and economic climate of the period, were not expected to appear anytime soon.[29] UNICEF leaders argued that such a model would ultimately strengthen district-level health systems in the long term by encouraging people to be self-reliant in terms of both labor and financing.[30] Introducing charges for health products and services was also supposed to spur people to make rational decisions about choosing care that they truly needed, thereby reducing extraneous or excess expenses. The Bamako Initiative thus combined the WHO's interest in building up primary health care with the interest of UNICEF and other agencies in decreasing dependence on states and external donors for health funding. While the politics behind these aims did not necessarily align, both were promoted under the guise of community ownership and empowerment.

President Moi signed the Bamako Initiative in 1987, thus displaying the country's political commitment to the policies of international donors. Kenya's Ministry of Health focused on extending basic health services to populations that had little access to government health facilities, by establishing community pharmacies that stocked a small selection of essential drugs, bed nets, and insecticide solution.[31] These pharmacies, located in some of the country's poorest areas, used initial inputs from UNICEF to obtain supplies and jump-start revolving fund schemes.[32] Kenya's Bamako Initiative projects advanced the government's health reforms and donors' desires under structural adjustment, filling gaps in the country's health infrastructure with markets.

UNICEF purchased considerable amounts of the supplies for Kenya's Bamako Initiative, building on its extensive experience with procuring health commodities for low-income countries. UNICEF representatives, however, did not consider the agency's procurement role as a permanent one. "Even with its broad-ranging and elastic mandate," a 1986 review of UNICEF activities stated, "UNICEF alone cannot provide most of the basic services to children and mothers in developing countries." Due to limited staff and the "relative weakness of its centers of operation," UNICEF operated better as "a supplementary force, a stimulus, a vehicle for experimentation, an added support."[33] UNICEF's imagined role fitted prevailing, supply-side approaches to health development at the time, whereby the availability of health goods would theoretically stimulate demand. Indeed, UNICEF representatives felt Bamako Initiative projects could teach people to value things such as immunizations and bed nets (particularly if a price were attached to these goods), which would in turn foster desire for them.[34] In providing seed supplies for Kenya's Bamako Initiative, UNICEF engaged this imaginary that supply and demand could sustain rural health care programs—an imaginary the World Bank, USAID, and other development agencies shared.

ITNs fit well with UNICEF's interest in using "affordable technology suited to the particular needs of rural and semi-urban areas," especially those tools that promoted child survival and maternal health.[35] Kiambo Njagi, a longtime member of the Ministry of Health and later the project coordinator for Kenya's National Malaria Control Program, remembered this congruence: "[The] Bamako Initiative came at the right time, because then, UNICEF was really interested in supporting mother and child. And therefore, a lot of nets and a lot of chemicals w[ere] distributed in Kenya through that method."[36] ITNs were also "well suited to community participation," a central component of UNICEF's plans to extend primary health care in Africa with limited financial and human resources.[37] ITNs became a material symbol of the government's commitment to the policy recommendations of international donors, on whom they relied to fund health activities in the country.

In September 1989, the Kenyan Ministry of Health and its partners initiated their first Bamako Initiative project in Kisumu district, followed shortly thereafter by projects in Homa Bay and Migori (all in what was formerly Nyanza Province). "Whenever you [went]" to the Bamako Initiative sites, Njagi recalled, you "could see a big jerry can of twenty liters of insecticide, bales of nets, and [a few] drugs in a very traditional hut."[38] Community health workers sold nets—most of which were imported from Thailand—for roughly US$3.30 to $4.20, charging US$0.50 for an insecticide dip.[39] Although it was a rather small sum, even the insecticide dip represented the monthly income of some of the poorest households served by these projects.[40] "From the beginning," explained one project reviewer, Kenya's Bamako Initiative scheme "has taken the view that in the interests of sustainability, neither nets nor insecticide would be distributed free of charge. This pricing strategy has the advantage of sending a clear message that the [insecticide-treated net] intervention involves two products, each of which has a price."[41] NGOs and research organizations extended Kenya's Bamako Initiative by initiating their own cost-recovery projects with ITNs, further decentralizing and privatizing health services and helping transform the Kenyan population into health consumers.[42]

Plans to establish self-sustaining, community-based primary health care services did not work as intended. Unsurprisingly, cost posed a major hindrance, especially when it came to re-dipping bed nets in insecticide. Roughly 33% of respondents in one study said cost was the reason they did not use bed nets from Bamako Initiative projects. And about 36% of those who did own nets were village leaders and others outside the target group of pregnant women and children, who were most at-risk for malaria.[43] Although pharmacies were supposed to help the poorest groups cover the cost of health products to address issues of equity, they struggled to maintain this assistance, especially since those areas with Bamako Initiative projects were more likely to serve some of the poorest populations. Some pharmacies could not make back enough money to reinvest in bed net supplies. Health workers at a project in West Pokot, for instance, offered loans to some people who could not afford bed nets but then faced significant challenges in collecting the loans once people had taken the nets home.[44] Many community pharmacies did not keep good records of sales and procurements, making it difficult to substantiate that those pharmacies actually made money on bed net sales.

Communities, moreover, did not operate as cohesively as policy makers had predicted. Largely male village health committees sometimes ran into conflicts with the mostly female community health workers who controlled the revenues from sales.[45] Such tensions underscore the observation that the use of "community" in descriptions of small-scale participatory projects often obscured the heterogeneity, power differentials, and constructed nature of intended beneficiary groups.[46] The program eventually petered out in 1996, when UNICEF stopped funding many of Kenya's Bamako Initiative projects.[47] This political vision of sustainable, low-cost health care in poor areas did not hold together in practice, though it continued to inform international discussions for disseminating ITNs in Africa during the 1990s.

Developing a Global Malaria Control Strategy in an Era of Scarcity

In 1992, as research teams and African health officials ramped up their investigations of insecticide-treated nets in both medical experiments and primary health care programs, the WHO aimed to put malaria back on the world health agenda. Specifically, the WHO planned to present its new Global Strategy for Malaria Control at a Global Ministerial Conference on Malaria. Securing greater political and financial commitment for malaria would be key elements of this presentation. In fact, the new strategy was not a detailed, prescriptive tool as much as a call for change cautiously undertaken by those in malaria-endemic countries and anyone else who could contribute resources to the effort. Early diagnosis and treatment remained the centerpiece of recommendations, despite rising rates of chloroquine resistance and a lack of affordable therapeutic alternatives. Planning and implementing "selective and sustainable preventive measures, including vector control," early detection and containment of epidemics, and strengthening local capabilities to assess a country's malaria situation—all open-ended, vague, or uncertain aims—rounded out the strategy's four technical elements.

The fact that the WHO moved ahead slowly with technical strategies while trying to drum up interest in malaria control was not lost on the agencies it hoped to court. "The document does not clearly communicate why, or how this 1992 strategy is different from approaches . . . taken in the 70's and 80's since the end of the eradication era," the USAID representative Dennis Carroll wrote about a draft of the strategy. "Nor is there a convincing argument made that if this strategy were implemented it would prove to be more effective than past strategies."[48] Given that the conference was "largely a media event," WHO representatives prepared to defend the new strategy to the international health and development community by preparing a list of answers to possible questions about the Ministerial Conference, including

"Why should residents of industrialized nations be concerned about malaria, if it is not a problem in their part of the country" and "Why did it take WHO and the UN Member States so long to change their policy from eradication to control?"[49] WHO officials knew they would be on the defensive as the organization sought to bring malaria to wider international attention.

The WHO's weak position relative to major donors created tension in malaria control policy during this era of resource scarcity: African states should do what was most suitable to their specific malaria situation, but only using those strategies sanctioned by groups with the necessary funds.[50] For instance, international health officials felt that health ministers of malaria-endemic countries should adopt the Global Malaria Control Strategy and adapt it to their own needs. David Nabarro, the chief health and population adviser at the UK Overseas Development Administration (later the Department for International Development [DFID]), reiterated that monolithic, world-scale plans for malaria control were not appropriate. The WHO's failed Malaria Eradication Programme had made that clear. Although countries needed to develop their own "realistic" control plans, however, Nabarro stressed that they also had to "develop programme proposals that cannot be refused by donors."[51] This meant that scientists and health officials in endemic countries had to produce knowledge about malaria control most likely to secure financial backing. Increasingly, such knowledge included calculations of medical efficacy—specifically the number of lives saved—and the cost-effectiveness of interventions.[52] Indeed, research teams measured these two metrics as main outcomes of their ITN trials over the subsequent years.

While ITNs did not figure prominently in the WHO's new global strategy, conference attendees, including leaders of WHO AFRO, promoted them unofficially as desirable health goods. Not all country representatives appreciated the WHO's new strategy or its promotion of ITNs. Dr. Timothy Stamps, Zimbabwe's minister of health and child welfare, opposed directives from the WHO concerning malaria control, arguing that they were inappropriate for his country. "We are advised to reduce our vector control programme without logical explanation," Stamps reported in his speech at the Ministerial Conference. "The achievable objective of controlling malaria transmission in agro-industrial estates in endemic areas is despised and the offer of unconventional inappropriate insecticide impregnated nets, with its immense logistical and health education problems is promoted through the appropriate commercial multi-national agencies."[53] Stamps also criticized the WHO for allowing the London-based Imperial Chemical Industries to advertise its ITN products at the conference, a sign of the organization's complicity in allowing commercial firms to profit from malaria prevention.[54]

Despite Stamps's criticisms, WHO AFRO's manager of disease prevention and control felt that the scarcity of resources for malaria control in Africa warranted support for the intervention. "Use of [insecticide-]impregnated bednets," he wrote, "is one of the few cost-efficient methods of malaria control in countries of high endemicity, which may be supported in a sustainable way. Therefore this intervention is encouraged by the WHO," despite the lack of knowledge about the technology's long-term effects. Regarding the presence of Imperial Chemical Industries, he continued, "it seems natural that companies promote their products. We think that excessively high price of bednets in Africa compared with Asia is the result of poor offer of the product." Competition in the bed net marketplace "might reduce the prices and make bednets affordable to the bulk of the African population."[55] With few other options, WHO AFRO officials embraced ITNs and called on African states to promote them, even though they had somewhat limited evidence for their effectiveness on the continent.

Amid this renewed international attention to malaria, Kenya's Ministry of Health developed the country's first National Plan of Action for Malaria Control in 1992. UNICEF and USAID supported the policy-making endeavor financially, sponsoring policy workshops and consultancies with American malaria experts.[56] Kenya's Ministry of Health used this plan to outline the state's commitment to malaria control and advocate the use of measures from the WHO's 1992 Global Malaria Control Strategy.[57] Establishing the government's commitment to sanctioned control methods was important since the ministry would require "substantial input" from donors to carry out the first two years of the plan.[58] The ministry also used the language of development to bolster support for its new national plan. "Malaria," Health Minister James Angatia wrote, "remains one of the most pressing health problems and impediments to social and economic development globally."[59] Malaria had a negative impact not only on people's health and survival but on "the country's economy and productivity as well."[60] The idea that health was a prerequisite for social and economic advancement resonated with major funding agencies, such as the World Bank and USAID, which prioritized economic development.[61]

Like its ongoing health care reform efforts, Kenya's National Plan of Action for Malaria Control reflected the country's commitment to the neoliberal principles of structural adjustment. Some of the plan's broad objectives included "improv[ing] and sustain[ing] community-based services for reducing malaria morbidity and mortality" and "empower[ing] community members to protect themselves from malaria related illness and death."[62] Again, the term "community-based" invoked the need for citizens to carry out and finance their own health interventions given the state's limited resources. The Ministry of Health included "personal protection measures," specifically ITNs, in the plan in pursuit of these goals. "The [Government of Kenya] will encourage communities to adopt the most appropriate technologies," the plan stated, in the case of insecticide-impregnated fabrics, the individual or collective dipping methods employed should be based on local customs, traditions, and preferences. Once a community has adopted the use of impregnated materials as an appropriate intervention, the [Ministry of Health] should encourage community members to sustain the programmes through cost-sharing."[63] As in Bamako Initiative projects, Kenyan health officials and their development agency partners imagined that Kenyan citizens would enact neoliberal health sector reforms by taking up ITNs.

While the Kenyan government continued to prioritize drug treatment in its 1992 National Plan of Action for Malaria Control, it also allocated money for the national dissemination of ITNs. Officials did this even before scientists had completed major randomized controlled efficacy trials with the intervention in the mid-1990s.[64] They did so in part to fulfill WHO AFRO's recommendation that member states adopt ITNs for "community-based" malaria control, even though WHO headquarters did not endorse the technology as strongly. Political imperatives to implement neoliberal health reforms under structural adjustment and the exigencies of curbing malaria on the cheap heavily informed Kenya's adoption of ITNs into health policy—more so than evidence of universal medical efficacy or directives from top-level international policy makers.

Envisioning ITN Implementation in a Neoliberal Era

Excitement about insecticide-treated nets continued to build following the 1992 Global Ministerial Conference, especially as research teams embarked on efficacy trials. Bed net treatment seemed simple and straightforward. African populations could treat nets at the village level, even in places without existing vector control programs.[65] While controlling malaria by preventing transmission (especially through indoor residual spraying campaigns) fell out of favor after the failure of malaria eradication in many countries, such an approach was "being re-considered using insecticide-treated nets . . . which do not require a large national programme infrastructure for implementation"—something that most African countries did not have and donors such as the World Bank actively opposed.[66] ITNs fitted political visions of public health and malaria control in Africa under structural adjustment, a quality that sometimes sidelined questions about the intervention's effectiveness or appropriateness in different settings.

However, malaria experts did not forget about the limitations and challenges of using ITNs in Africa during this period. Two members of the WHO Malaria Unit, Pierre Carnevale and Awash Teklehaimanot, noted that the technology would not be very efficacious in situations where vectors were exophilic (fed outdoors) or zoophagic (fed mainly on nonhuman animals), and where people slept outdoors. It would also be difficult to implement the intervention in places where, for "financial and cultural reasons," people were not already using bed nets.[67] Since studies showed that African populations could describe the benefits of using ITNs and still decide not to use the tool, they reiterated that "there is no single solution applicable everywhere with the same expected efficacy."[68] Producing further knowledge about the biomedical efficacy or cost-effectiveness of ITNs could not overcome some limitations of using the technology to curb malaria on the continent.

These same experts also conceived possible plans to overcome the challenges of implementing ITNs on a large scale in Africa. Some suggestions, such as providing nets at a "reasonable price" and using targeted health education, proved too simplistic in practice.[69] Other proposals were more ambitious, such as creating provincial bed net centers that could "serve as a focal point for promoting bednets, providing training in impregnation, and assuring the supply of bednets and insecticides," and "promote community participation in malaria control activities in general."[70] While these alternative plans imagined a somewhat more robust infrastructure of community-based health care than plans to sell nets through retail outlets, they similarly reflected the broader decentralization of health systems on the continent.

Confident that ITNs would eventually take off, members of the Special Programme for Research and Training in Tropical Diseases (TDR) and others who had worked on bed net projects convened an international meeting about the intervention in November 1994. The meeting was held in Dar es Salaam, Tanzania, a country that since the early 1980s had been the site of substantial bed net testing—both in terms of the intervention's effectiveness for malaria control and its viability in community-based programs. Christian Lengeler, Jacqueline Cattani, and Don de Savigny compiled conversations from this meeting into a book, *Net Gain: A New Method for Preventing Malaria Deaths*. As the book describes, experiences from small-scale bed net implementation projects—including Kenya's Bamako Initiative scheme—did not provide models for successful and sustainable programs as much as they elucidated pitfalls and questions.[71] Therefore, the authors called for more effectiveness studies of ITNs, which would provide knowledge on how best to scale up the intervention on the continent.

This 1994 meeting generated many lines of thinking about the practicality of implementing ITNs. However, it catalyzed one development in particular: at this conference, participants considered social marketing as a desirable distribution method. In short, social marketing applies concepts and tools from commercial marketing to a socially beneficial product or behavior (such as those associated with public health). Social marketing agencies, for example, often use market research techniques to brand products and sell them at highly subsidized prices to teach people about the product's health benefits. Theoretically, people will also learn to value and desire the product. By selling such goods in pharmacies, retail outlets, and, less commonly, clinics, social marketers aim to transfer the burden of health care provision from the public to the private sector. The government and external donors can then focus their resources on helping the poorest populations. In many ways, social marketing embodied the increasingly neoliberal character of international health.

Although those working on ITN projects in the mid-1990s may have been unfamiliar with social marketing at that point, the method was by no means new. During the 1970s USAID began investing heavily in social marketing projects for contraceptives as part of its broader support for supply-side approaches to family planning. Leveraging the "flexibility and innovativeness of the private sector," the agency aimed to distribute efficiently and stimulate demand for birth control in low-income countries.[72] USAID contracted with private voluntary organizations such as Population Services International (PSI) to do this work.[73] Even though social marketing projects had limited success in reducing birth rates, USAID continued to invest in the method for other health interventions, such as oral rehydration salts to treat dehydration and condoms for HIV/AIDS prevention. DFID and other development agencies followed USAID's lead in the 1990s, seeking to make health care in low-income countries more efficient and less dependent on external donors, by tapping into the private sector.

Perceived successes with some of these social marketing projects, particularly condom distribution in Africa during the late 1980s and early 1990s, inspired attempts to use the approach for ITNs. Conference attendees thought that social marketing might be especially useful for convincing people to treat their nets with insecticide regularly, which few participants in pilot programs did either because they did not understand the insecticide's benefits or believe that the treatment was worth the cost and hassle. "At that conference, there was a guy called Tim Manchester . . . working in Dar es Salaam for a group called PSI," de Savigny recalled,

> and they were social marketing condoms all over Africa. And he heard about our meeting up at Kunduchi Beach hotel and started clamoring to be part of it. And we didn't know him. It was all bed net people. And we didn't know anything about social marketing. And he said, "I want to talk on the agenda. I want to talk about social marketing." . . . And so we said, "okay, you can have fifteen minutes. We'll squeeze you in." We had a pretty full program. And he got up, and it went for about an hour, hour-and-a-half. It was incredibly fascinat[ing]. Everyone was riveted. And [that] was the moment where we said, "ah, this was our way out. This was our way forward. This is how we're gonna get past this problem of dipping nets." . . . What he said actually was a route that we started to take.[74]

This concern with getting people to treat their bed nets with insecticide—an issue that threatened the ability of the technology to prevent malaria or save lives—also spawned new innovations that made social marketing seem more feasible. During the mid-1990s Jane Miller, who had worked on bed net research in Tanzania, developed a home treatment kit for her doctoral dissertation project with the London School of Hygiene and Tropical Medicine (LSHTM). Recognizing that people could not always access communal dipping sites either for reasons of poor geographic access or inability to afford treatment services during the period that they were offered, Miller and her colleagues introduced an individual insecticide sachet (similar to a pod of laundry soap) paired with a set of disposable gloves. People could use these in the privacy of their own homes to dip bed nets, much as they would wash clothes. The home treatment kit obviated the need for mass dipping services, which were complicated as well as inconvenient. As "a product that could be sold in small shops alongside [mosquito] coils and sprays, and that could be used safely and effectively even by inexperienced and untrained people," the kits also served as a tangible way for health programmers to sell the task of re-treating nets to African populations.[75] Miller took her home treatment kit to PSI, then the largest social marketing agency in the world and the first to become involved with ITNs. The kit would eventually make its way into a variety of social marketing projects and programs on the continent. Donors' political and economic interests, as well as the material forms of the intervention, played a significant role in decisions about how best to distribute ITNs on the continent.

Translating Research into Policy

As the preceding sections make clear, health officials and program leaders working in Africa were not waiting for randomized controlled trial evidence to proceed with insecticide-treated net activities. This does not mean that scientific findings played little or no role in the policy-making process. Scientists wrapped up the four TDR-sponsored bed net trials around 1995–1996, the results of which had fueled new enthusiasm for the technology. "There's never been an intervention that's had such a huge effect on under-five mortality," de Savigny told me. "And our back of the envelope calculations on cost-effectiveness put it right down in there in the range of immunizations, and so on. So we knew we had a winner."[76] Advocates, including many scientists who had worked on the ITN trials, mobilized experimental results to convince major donors to invest in the intervention and malaria control in Africa more generally. This helped elevate nets as a main element of global malaria control policy by the late 1990s, especially as policy makers knew they would need to recommend strategies likely to attract donor support.

The work of advocates was important because scientific findings alone did not catalyze widespread support for ITNs. People outside TDR did not initially share scientists' excitement about the randomized controlled trials. Christian Lengeler remembered sharing preliminary trial results with people at WHO headquarters in 1995, but they were "absolutely not interested."[77] Research teams also tried to publish results from the trials together in the *Lancet*, a highly influential journal that could sway opinion on the acceptance of health interventions, but the journal did not take them.[78] "Back then," de Savigny continued,

> Lancet was a medical journal, and a preventive intervention that was a non-vaccine or a non-drug was not interesting. It didn't matter the public health power of this intervention. . . . And they [Lancet editors] said, "Well, you know, a few years ago Steve Lindsay and Greenwood and Bob Snow published [results from the Gambian mortality trial]. . . . We know bed nets save lives. Big deal." And so it was rejected. And we lost six months, the world lost six months. You add up how many children died in a six-month period from malaria, this is a consequence of not being able to talk out loud about a publishable result.[79]

They eventually published their results in 1996 in *Tropical Medicine and International Health*. Yet even then, it took a while for the international community to commit to providing any significant resources for ITNs in Africa. Robust scientific results of efficacy and cost-effectiveness by themselves did not translate immediately into policy action.

Still, experimental findings demonstrating that ITNs could reduce child mortality were critical to legitimizing the technology for malaria control in Africa, an endeavor many donors "wr[o]te-off" as a potential waste of money in previous decades.[80] "We did go through an incredibly dry phase from the end of the global malaria eradication programme through to the 80s of making malaria a far less specialized thing," Bob Snow recalled.

> It became embedded in primary health care. No one had a malaria thing that they could then pursue. And then bed nets actually became that. It became a malaria specific intervention. . . . It became the champion of all the trials. They were fabulous results. And . . . it's not right to say, as people were saying, "Well we don't know what to do." Actually, then we could say, "We do know what to do." And there were two things we could do: to treat malaria properly with the right drug and put a child—or as many household members as you could—under an insecticide-treated bed net. And that was perfect because that's all donors needed. They needed to know that it was simple, and . . . they only need two things, and [they] could afford it. And I think that transformed everything.[81]

On top of that, members of TDR claimed, findings from the recent efficacy trials "emphasized the underestimated contribution of malaria to child mortality in Africa and the potentially large benefits of malaria-preventive interventions."[82] The trials provided the proof of concept necessary to show that controlling malaria helped accomplish the international health and development goals of saving children's lives in a cost-effective way.

ITN advocates in and outside Africa continued to drum up support by holding meetings where they called on others to commit resources to the implementation of WHO-sanctioned strategies. After many years of discussing the need for malaria control, the WHO director-general, Hiroshima Nakajima, committed $20 million for the "Accelerated Implementation of Malaria Control" in thirty-four African countries. Malaria experts hoped that this exercise would lay a foundation for national malaria control programs and give donors confidence that African countries could make progress in controlling the disease with the necessary inputs.[83] At times, selling malaria control as a good investment and establishing political commitment to the cause appeared to be an end in itself rather than a means to an end.

Despite these efforts, African leaders remained frustrated by the continued lack of resources for malaria control. In June 1997 the Organization of African Unity met for its thirty-third ordinary session in Harare, Zimbabwe. Participating African leaders adopted the Harare Declaration on Malaria Prevention and Control in the Context of African Economic Recovery and Development, restating their commitment to malaria control and to the WHO's Global and Regional Malaria Control Strategies. After years of bringing malaria into the limelight, however, many national programs were still just beginning to implement malaria interventions. While tools for malaria control that could reduce deaths and illness in Africa were available, they were "not accessible, for various reasons, in appropriate forms."[84] The Organization of African Unity called on the private sector and NGOs, along with multi- and bilateral agencies to provide technical and financial resources for malaria control, though they hoped such efforts would "build a foundation for sustainable malaria control" and not become a temporary patch for the problem. At the same time, the organization called on African leaders and health officials to support microfinancing schemes for malaria control projects and "sensitize" populations to adopt personal protection measures, including mosquito nets, which could be carried out by families and communities.[85]

In late 1997 major donor agencies finally consolidated support for ITNs. Riding a wave of US Senate support for global infectious disease control, the USAID representative Dennis Carroll convened an International Conference on Bednets and Other Insecticide-Treated Materials in Washington, DC, in October of that year.[86] It was at this conference that Christian Lengeler presented a meta-analysis of all the ITN efficacy trials, excluding the ongoing trial in Siaya discussed in chapter 2. For Lengeler, this was where researchers "won the war of making the results known and getting [the] interest of all the big guys at the time."[87] Funding agencies "are a little bit reluctant to take on new things, but if they see that their neighbors think it's a good idea, then suddenly the interest is much stronger."[88]

Getting donors on board had its trade-offs, however, as donors prioritized certain concerns over others. Even though Carroll invited public health practitioners to participate in this conference, the organizers did not intend that the conference deal with the technical aspects of ITNs as a public health measure, such as the need for strong health information systems—which many African countries did not have—or questions about how high ITN coverage would have to be to affect malaria levels. While such unresolved issues had great relevance for ensuring the effectiveness of nets as a public health measure, the conference instead focused on figuring out ways to get African "consumers and potential consumers" to accept, desire, purchase, and use ITNs.[89] Development agencies with the resources needed to disseminate ITNs approached the technology as a commercial product that could succeed in Africa with precise marketing research, appropriate communication, and strong market-based distribution systems. In the process, they took for granted how the tool affected mosquitoes, environments, and other malaria control activities.

Promoting Roll Back Malaria and ITNs

In 1998 the incoming director-general of the WHO, Gro Harlem Brundtland, tapped into wealthy countries' new interest in insecticide-treated nets and malaria control and established the Roll Back Malaria program. The WHO, World Bank, UNICEF, and United Nations Development Programme jointly sponsored the program, which Brundtland conceived of as an experiment and model for major public-private partnerships across the WHO.[90] She hoped that Roll Back Malaria could make the case for including health activities in development priorities, stressing the impediment malaria posed to both economic progress and good health in Africa and the global south.[91] Brundtland received support for Roll Back Malaria from the leaders of major industrialized countries at the 1998 G8 Summit in Birmingham in the name of helping African countries better integrate into the global economy.[92] Critical of the WHO's ability to raise and use funds effectively, the

World Bank in particular felt that a public-private partnership like Roll Back Malaria would be more likely to sustain malaria control activities.[93] Brundtland and her colleagues at the WHO used Roll Back Malaria to assert the continued relevance of the organization, as the World Bank surpassed the WHO as the leading patron of international health activities.[94]

Although the program specifically targeted malaria, Brundtland sold Roll Back Malaria as an endeavor to build up and reform the health sectors of malaria-endemic countries. "Rolling Back Malaria," she told the World Health Assembly in May 1998, "is no victory unless health systems are equipped to sustain the gains."[95] Initial plans for Roll Back Malaria therefore included promoting health system decentralization and developing community-based health financing mechanisms.[96] On these grounds, Brundtland touted Roll Back Malaria as something new that was more than just "a revamped vertical programme," reminiscent of the WHO's failed, top-down eradication campaign.[97] David Nabarro, Roll Back Malaria's first executive director, articulated a similar vision, claiming that the program would not use a "one fit-all" solution for malaria, but rather help develop African health systems, improve health education, and "adapt basic strategies . . . so that they respond to people's needs within the limits of resources available in their societies."[98] Nabarro's statement also reflected the priorities of DFID, his home institution and Roll Back Malaria's largest funder during its early years, which sought to build local capacity so aid recipients could sustain activities after donors withdrew support.[99]

Despite such emphases on the program's novelty, Roll Back Malaria inherited most of its technical strategies from earlier malaria control policies. Rapid diagnosis and treatment, disease prevention, and early detection of epidemics remained central pillars. Since ITNs had garnered significant attention as disease prevention measures, Roll Back Malaria policy makers recommended the intervention as a main strategy. In doing so, they constituted ITNs as a tangible and countable means by which private sector, NGO, and development agency partners could contribute to the fight against malaria.

An important element in Brundtland's plan to attract financial resources for malaria and other public health causes was to present decision makers with "solid evidence."[100] Statistical results and measurable goals were key. Scientists believed that ITNs had the evidence base required for securing scarce resources, which were overwhelmingly dedicated to HIV/AIDS at the time. Lengeler published his meta-analysis of ITN trial results—also known as a Cochrane Review—in May 1998, around the same time Brundtland proposed Roll Back Malaria to the World Health Assembly.[101] Many felt that Lengeler's Cochrane Review offered "conclusive proof" of the biomedical efficacy of ITNs.[102] "Most Cochrane Reviews, to be honest, say 'we need more data' as the concluding comment," Bob Snow told me. "This one didn't. You don't need more data. This is pretty [good] evidence that it reduces morbidity, it reduces child mortality. Also, because we looked at this, it reduces hospitalization for malaria. You can reduce the incidence of anemia. This is fantastic. I think the pooled analysis showed that you could reduce all-cause childhood mortality by about seventeen percent. And there was nothing else out there—not an immunization strategy, not a clean water sort of thing—could have that size of an effect."[103] Clinical epidemiology and biostatistics transformed ITNs into proxies for lives saved, making them competitive in the marketplace of health and development interventions.[104]

Of course, as someone personally involved in bed net studies in various capacities, Lengeler recognized the gap between efficacy trial results and the effectiveness of ITN programs. The Medical Research Council's experience in The Gambia revealed that getting people to pay to regularly re-treat nets with insecticide presented an especially difficult obstacle.[105] Lengeler and many others agreed that malaria control programmers needed more data on ITN effectiveness outside controlled experimental conditions. He also noted in his Cochrane Review that the efficacy of ITNs in high-risk areas—an issue scientists were investigating in Siaya at the time—remained uncertain. Others articulated similar reservations, questioning whether nets would interfere with other malaria control methods or be suitable in places where vectors had already started to become resistant to pyrethroids.[106] Lengeler nevertheless felt that questions about long-term impact should not impede the dissemination of ITNs during the ongoing malaria crisis. "Given the strength of this evidence," he reported, "there is a need to promote the large-scale application of this tool."[107]

And, even given the "fantastic results" from bed net trials, policy makers did not limit their recommendations for malaria prevention measures to ITNs alone, at least on paper. Roll Back Malaria policy makers called on African heads of state to help at-risk populations "benefit from the most suitable combination of personal and community protective measures such as insecticide treated mosquito nets and other interventions which are accessible and affordable to prevent infection and suffering."[108] These interventions included house screening, environmental management, and other measures that fit into decentralized health systems. In practice, however, these other methods did not figure into assessments of African malaria control programs or attract financial support. Environmental management, house screening, and mosquito repellent did not have the scientific markers of a lifesaving, "evidence-based" intervention that ITNs did. Without confidence regarding the health impact provided by randomized controlled trial results, donors would not invest in such activities.

Lack of efficacy data for these other prevention measures also meant that health economists could not provide the cost-effectiveness calculations "needed for the WHO Roll Back Malaria campaign."[109] An increased desire for econometrics to rationalize investments in international health during this period significantly circumscribed approaches to malaria control in Africa. "The lack of data," economists from LSHTM reported, "precluded analysis of several potentially important interventions, including environmental management, epidemic surveillance and prevention, and interventions to improve the treatment of severe malaria."[110] ITNs thus possessed attributes other than biomedical efficacy that led to their adoption as a central tool for global malaria control. As one of the most cost-effective malaria prevention measures for very low-income countries—and one of the few with any cost-effectiveness data—ITNs attracted much of the attention from donors and, thus, policy makers.

The tension between what health officials thought would be beneficial and what they promoted based on the exigencies of fundraising emerged yet again. Recalling outcries against the failure of one-size-fits-all approaches, Roll Back Malaria leaders claimed that participating state governments should tailor program recommendations to their specific national circumstances. Yet all national malaria programs were supposed to track the percentage of children under five sleeping under an ITN.[111] In fact, although Roll Back Malaria leaders originally set a target of 60% coverage of at-risk populations with "suitable" disease prevention measures, they only planned to track coverage of intermittent presumptive treatment for pregnant women and ITNs to measure the program's progress. They did not even plan to track intermittent presumptive treatment everywhere since some places lacked the necessary antimalarial drugs. Measuring progress toward coverage goals alongside malaria disease indicators would demonstrate impact to donors eager to make a return on their investments. Roll Back Malaria leaders believed that when donor agencies saw this impact they would in turn be convinced to continue supporting malaria control both financially and politically.

With nominal support from wealthy countries and development agencies, Roll Back Malaria assumed authority over worldwide malaria control. This leadership transition reinforced gaps in knowledge about how best to disseminate ITNs in Africa, especially since the partnership focused on co-ordinating activities and convincing donors to invest in the cause. "So Roll Back Malaria was created in '98," de Savigny recounted, "and of course [insecticide-treated nets] became a big, big chunk of [Roll Back Malaria's] effort, correctly. And so TDR looked at that when we were trying to say, 'We have to do this implementation research,' and said, 'Oh, no, that actually is [Roll Back Malaria's] job now.' And then we went to [Roll Back Malaria] and said, 'Well, no, that's research. That's TDR's job.' . . . TDR . . . [ellipsis in the original] no guts to say, 'We have to now do the "how" questions.' This hand-off never occurred."[112] Randomized controlled trials may have helped render ITNs as universally applicable biomedical technologies that worked the same way in every local context. But they did not accomplish this transformation on their own. The momentum of the policy-making and fundraising process, in which efficacy and cost-effectiveness statistics played a key role, left many questions about the intervention unanswered and seemingly irrelevant to those capable of funding malaria programming.

When it came time to guide African countries on how to scale up ITNs, Roll Back Malaria officials gravitated toward social marketing. In 1999 they commissioned a "Strategic Plan for ITN Social Marketing" from PSI/Europe, sponsored by DFID. Citing PSI's experience with running social marketing programs for family planning and AIDS prevention, officials called on the agency to identify strategies for product and brand positioning, distribution, promotion, behavior change communications, and social mobilization.[113] In moving forward with this social marketing approach, they further rendered ITNs as products whose essential, biomedical utility and value simply had to be revealed to intended users, even though scientists knew from their experiments that African populations often did not internalize or prioritize this value. This also continued to divert attention away from technical questions, such as what level of ITN coverage was appropriate in different epidemiological settings.[114]

Roll Back Malaria's promotion of ITNs attracted support from a variety of organizations, not all of which were familiar with the outstanding technical questions about the intervention. For instance, they communicated with the US development group Crown Agents Ltd., which offered its services in negotiating bulk purchases of nets and chemicals from manufacturers. "We are aware that a major part of [Roll Back Malaria] is the provision of insecticide treated bednets (ITN's) which are such a simple yet effective way of preventing malaria thus potentially saving millions of lives," wrote the director of procurement sales and marketing, David Jamieson. "This initiative of course depends on the availability of good quality nets at an affordable price and in the quantities required to deliver optimum results," an availability Jamieson thought that Crown Agents could help achieve.[115]

Just as cost-effectiveness calculations and randomized controlled trial results helped create equivalencies between ITNs and vaccines or pharmaceuticals via cost per life saved, marketing groups compared and equated ITNs with other health commodities. "The impact of the [Roll Back Malaria] Programme on the market for bednets," Jamieson continued, "has many similarities to the affects [sic] on the demand for male latex condoms after Cairo [International Conference on Population and Development] and in response to the HIV/AIDS pandemic." Therefore, he claimed, Roll Back Malaria partners should look to experiences with condom supply and demand to strengthen social marketing with ITNs.[116] As Roll Back Malaria leaders sought to attract patrons and partners to the cause of malaria control in Africa, appealing to these groups' interests and expertise in using markets to deliver public health goods, they further obscured the contingencies and complexities of ITNs.

Making Evidence-Based Policy in Kenya

On April 25, 2000, heads of state and other delegates from forty-four African countries met in Abuja, Nigeria, for the first African Summit on Roll Back Malaria. Country representatives signed the Abuja Declaration at the meeting, pledging to commit themselves to the goals and approaches of Roll Back Malaria. These goals included halving malaria mortality by 2010 using prompt diagnosis and treatment, insecticide-treated nets, and intermittent presumptive therapy for pregnant women. More specifically, signatories agreed to strive for 60% coverage of at-risk populations—defined as pregnant women and children under five—with these interventions by 2005. By signing the declaration, African leaders also agreed to allocate the resources required to carry out Roll Back Malaria activities in their respective countries and waive taxes and tariffs on imported bed nets and insecticides.[117] In exchange for committing their countries to the program, governments would benefit from debt relief granted by development agency partners. In addition, they put themselves in a position to receive aid for malaria control activities from private, academic, NGO, and other bilateral partners that joined Roll Back Malaria—aid increasingly tied to ITNs.

President Moi signed the Abuja Declaration, pledging to incorporate Roll Back Malaria strategies into Kenya's national malaria control activities.[118] In contrast to the Bamako Initiative, which targeted multiple health problems in poor, rural areas, this public health financing strategy focused on a specific disease target and explicit national-level disease control measures. Even with the new sources, scale, and organization of funding, however, the decentralized, privatized strategies for ITN distribution characteristic of Bamako Initiative projects remained intact.

Kenyan health officials did not adopt Roll Back Malaria strategies overnight.[119] Once the WHO had announced the program's launch in 1998, members of Kenya's National Malaria Control Programme and Kenya Medical Research Institute/Wellcome Trust began preparing to implement Roll Back Malaria recommendations. They conducted a situation analysis outlining the extent of malaria in Kenya as well as the existing malaria control activities, partners, and projects in the country, which provided a picture of what health officials had to work with.[120] This situation analysis signaled the growing dominance of ITNs in global malaria control: whereas Kenya's previous malaria control policies recommended an array of personal protection measures, the authors of this situation analysis narrowed their discussion to ITNs specifically. Nets, after all, had an extremely positive Cochrane Review to their name.

Kenya's experience with adopting ITNs, though, showed that scientific evidence did not always drive disease control policy. "It is notable," the authors of the situation analysis wrote, "that efforts to introduce this preventative strategy in 1990 begun [sic] before the definitive clinical trials were completed in 1995. Thus providing an example of where research is not always required before policy recommendation."[121] For the authors, clinical trials also did not resolve important operational questions. "Whilst there is a growing trend toward [insecticide-treated bed net] promotion and distribution[,] more imaginative and appropriate delivery approaches must be explored to improve coverage."[122] Getting people to re-treat bed nets—an obstacle that health officials encountered in Bamako Initiative projects—was particularly important if this intervention was to have "a demonstrable impact on child survival."[123] Health programmers in Kenya recognized the uphill battle they faced in reaching Roll Back Malaria goals for ITN coverage well before President Moi signed the Abuja Declaration.

Kenya's Ministry of Health, technical advisers (notably Bob Snow), and members of donor agencies met to prepare a national malaria control strategy over the following two years in line with Roll Back Malaria strategies. Since the Kenyan government needed to mobilize substantial external resources for malaria control, state health officials had to engage with the interests, priorities, and ideas of multiple international partners and potential contributors. The head of the newly created Division of Malaria Control, Sam Ochola, and his colleagues described this as "a process of selecting evidence-based approaches, broad stakeholder participation and harmonisation with the National Health Sector Strategic Plan."[124] Behind the scenes, this was difficult to do. It "was an interesting departure for me," Snow remembered, "because I was a hardcore scientist who had never had to work within a political arena with people who had their own opinions on how things should be done, and . . . at that time, [were] less concerned about evidence, more concerned about what they used to do."[125] Developing an "evidence-based" malaria control policy had as much to do with political negotiation as translating scientific findings into a plan of action.

As Ochola, Snow, and others learned through this process, donors had tremendous influence on how to integrate ITNs into national policy since they were the ones putting up the necessary resources. "There were those hardcore advocates for private sector delivery of bed nets, and there were those like myself," Snow told me, "who thought it should all be free. . . . We ended up coming up with a structure of an enabling environment, and everyone would have a piece of the pie, knowing full well, of course, that those who had the money to do things only ended up doing them. That was social marketing at the time."[126] Furthermore, not all donors agreed on how to do things. Snow continued, "USAID, DFID, DANIDA—everyone had their own agenda. . . . I was someone completely independent. And the Director of Medical Services at the time actually felt that that was a useful contribution for him to have someone that was independent and could just tell donors, 'Look, frankly, your contribution to this strategy is a fleet of Toyota land cruisers. Actually, that's not what we need.' Where it's harder for the Director of Medical Services to say that from a political point of view."[127] Tailoring Roll Back Malaria recommendations to Kenya's specific situation—the stated aim of the new global strategy—meant in large part negotiating the competing interests of those entities that were able to fund malaria control activities.

Partly for this reason, PSI came to play a major role in Kenya's effort to scale up ITNs nationally, despite the social marketing agency's less-than-stellar track record in pilot projects. In 1997 PSI had carried out a social marketing project with ITNs in Kilifi.[128] Since most residents already had nets from the recent randomized controlled trial, PSI focused on getting people to re-treat their nets. Just four months after PSI introduced a cost-retrieval system for insecticide treatment in Kilifi, coverage of net re-treatment dropped from about 60% to 7%.[129] More than 80% of mothers who did not bring their child's net for re-treatment claimed that they could not afford the service, priced at 25 Kenyan shillings (less than US$1 at the time). "Community financing mechanisms described in Tanzania (Makemba et al. 1995) and The Gambia (Mills et al. 1994)," researchers claimed, "require established village or community structures not well defined among the scattered settlement populations along the Kenyan Coast."[130] Those analyzing the project added that "food often t[ook] priority over other expenditures for the limited household cash resources."[131] Like earlier Bamako Initiative projects, PSI's experience in Kilifi illustrated the difficulty of getting poor populations in the country to take up ITNs.

Nevertheless, social marketing fitted donors' desires to transfer more of the burden of health care provision to the private and nongovernmental sectors. "Social marketing was the happy comprise by many to say that, 'well, we'll make poor people pay a bit and then they'll value it and we will create that long term net culture,'" Bob Snow recalled. "I think all the evidence we had accumulated in Kenya, at least, [showed] they were all absolute failures in reaching coverage levels that were needed to impact transmission and make a dent in malaria mortality."[132] Although Kenyan health officials invited many partners to the table to help craft the country's malaria control strategy, collaboration had its limits. According to one policy document, PSI "did not participate fully during the early consensus building exercise but rather preferred to present the social marketing case directly to the Deputy Director

of Medical Services."[133] Evidence from Kenya did not support social marketing, but donor funding did.

Kenya's government continued to play a role in national malaria control
activities, but this role largely entailed facilitating the creation of markets for
ITNs. Following recommendations from Roll Back Malaria partners, the
government agreed to lower taxes and tariffs on ITN products to reflect
their new "public health value."[134] The Ministry of Health would also oversee the regulation of commodities and funding of information, education,
and communication activities to help create demand for bed nets and insecticide.[135] They took on this role, not because market mechanisms proved
particularly effective at disseminating ITNs in Kenya, but because they
needed resources from many external organizations that supported market-
based approaches. In this donor-dominated process of evidence-based policy
making, only certain aspects of ITNs—namely, their biomedical efficacy
and cost-effectiveness—seemed to require substantive demonstrations of
proof. The politics of public health did not.

Scientists and health officials came to understand ITNs as an evidence-based
intervention by the end of the twentieth century. Policy makers mobilized
this status to justify including the technology as a centerpiece in the new Roll
Back Malaria program. Looking at the history of malaria control policy in the
post-eradication period, however, complicates the idea that statistics of biomedical efficacy and cost-effectiveness calculations—the gold standard of
evidence—alone dictated this development. For example, African health officials sometimes adopted ITNs in national health policies and programs before scientists showed that the intervention could reduce child mortality or
agreed that they were effective in diverse epidemiological settings. This was
the case in Kenya, where state health officials first disseminated nets in a
primary health care program that made citizens more responsible for operating and financing their own health services, especially in areas that were
underserved by government health resources. This program and Kenya's 1992
National Plan of Action for Malaria Control were components of the government's larger effort to implement structural adjustment reforms under
pressure from the World Bank and other donors. ITNs appeared well-suited
to the new system, which prioritized decentralizing and privatizing the health
sector. They thus became a tool for securing much needed resources and sup-

port from external funders. ITNs served not only as a symbol but also as a technology of neoliberal policy.

WHO officials, including leaders of WHO AFRO, similarly leveraged the suitability of ITNs for cost-effective, community-based health care to secure financial support for malaria control from donors during the 1990s. ITNs provided a way to curb malaria in Africa without building centralized public health infrastructure or investing in substantial technical and human resources, which many major development agencies did not want to do. When WHO leaders launched Roll Back Malaria in 1998, they not only championed nets as a main pillar of malaria control but did so within a broader framework of decentralizing and privatizing health systems in Africa. In the new neoliberal regime of "global health" symbolized by the public-private partnership, ITNs did not simply function as malaria control devices; they also served as tools for reforming African health sectors and transforming citizens into private consumers of public health goods.

The entwined political and scientific character of ITNs had significant consequences for global malaria control. Randomized controlled trial results together with politically popular social marketing approaches and gaps in operational research worked to obscure the complexities of ITNs as malaria control tools. In their plans to disseminate the intervention, donor agencies and their private sector and nongovernmental partners only considered statistical results from efficacy trials. They did not account for the various contingencies that affected the technology's ability to save children's lives, which scientists and health officers had learned about in experiments and pilot projects. The reduction of ITNs to their biomedical use value, or their ability to save lives in any setting, underwrote development agencies' plans to deliver the tool using private and nongovernmental channels. At the same time, such reductionism allowed these donors to equate and compare ITNs with other lifesaving interventions in the "global health economy," a favorable comparison for the relatively cheap, low-tech product.[136] Health policy makers and scientist-advocates of malaria control, therefore, marshaled data on the efficacy and cost-effectiveness of ITNs not only to claim that the object was a useful tool for curbing malaria in Africa but also to sell malaria control as a worthy investment in the twenty-first century.

4

The Global Health Commodity

Selling the Value of Saving Lives

In 1999 NetMark, a project dedicated solely to scaling up insecticide-treated nets, joined a growing roster of organizations that had signed up to roll back malaria in Africa. Funded by the United States Agency for International Development (USAID), NetMark reveals much about the state of global malaria control at the dawn of the twenty-first century. This private sector health initiative worked with commercial manufacturers and local distributors to expand the market for ITNs in Africa. It sought to develop this market not only by increasing insecticide and bed net supplies but also by using behavior change communication and marketing techniques to foster consumer demand on the continent. The United States and other wealthy countries found this private sector approach appealing because they felt it would require less input from governments and external donors in the long run and be more efficient than public sector delivery models. USAID's assistant administrator for global health, Anne Peterson, was so confident in the benefits of private sector partnerships that she predicted for the US Congress that a venture like NetMark would "serve as a model in other parts of the world and with other health related products."[1] Finally, NetMark and USAID justified their limited focus on distributing ITNs to control malaria by citing the technology's ability to "cut all-cause child mortality by 17–63%" with consistent use even in "desperately poor countries."[2] Valuing ITNs for their ability to save lives in the context of scarce resources, NetMark and its sponsors facilitated the widespread circulation of this tool in a competitive economy of global health interventions.

NetMark's creation was enmeshed in two trends in twenty-first-century global health: the rise of public-private partnerships and the privileging of "evidence-based" interventions. These trends converged in global malaria control efforts to perpetuate a narrow focus on ITN distribution, even as Roll Back Malaria leaders touted their horizontal, nationally tailored approach to the disease. Statistical evidence from clinical trials, cited by Dr. Peterson, construed ITNs as tangible proxies for lives saved. As individual-use technologies, these objects also appeared to fit well into capitalist systems, where the levers of supply and demand could be manipulated to deliver social and economic benefits. Wealthy donors concerned with measuring the impact of their investments, or "accountability," found both aspects attractive. Starting in 1998, Roll Back Malaria leaders capitalized on these groups' enthusiasm for ITNs to attract new resources and partners for malaria control in Africa, linking the saving of lives to humanitarian and economic goals.[3] The need to demonstrate success to attract further financial support created a feedback loop that encouraged African countries to distribute ITNs as quickly as possible, with little regard for the contingencies and labor required to make nets work as malaria control devices. This process helped cement ITNs' identity as standardized goods, procured and circulated through international markets and local distribution channels based on a simplified conception of their ability to save lives cost-effectively. In other words, this process reified them as global health commodities.[4]

This chapter examines how African countries and their external partners scaled up ITNs under Roll Back Malaria. This process not only depended on ITNs' emergent identity as global health commodities—which donors procured to save lives and promote economic development across widely different contexts—but also reinforced this identity. Roll Back Malaria served as a fundraiser, coordinator, and advocate for malaria control activities, uniting diverse groups and interests around a common technical strategy. At times, its leaders put their need to sustain and grow the partnership before the need to implement the most effective approaches, the former seen as a prerequisite for the latter. Since many donors preferred ITNs as a solution for malaria in Africa, African countries that joined Roll Back Malaria largely received net-related support regardless of whether this was the most useful or appropriate intervention for their specific circumstances.[5] Calls to increase funding for malaria control translated into more and more ITNs.

New global health governance and funding mechanisms may have rendered ITNs as global health commodities, but the nets' identity as cost-effective, lifesaving goods did not always hold together on the ground. Based on their prior experiences with ITN distribution as well as donor preferences, different African countries relied on different, sometimes piecemeal strategies for scaling up the intervention. Many of these strategies, especially those that relied on selling nets and insecticide, were not very successful in increasing ITN coverage. Target consumers did not always buy or use the intervention as program leaders and donors had intended. Although children under five and pregnant women, especially those living in poor rural areas, were considered the most at risk for malaria, their families often could not afford ITNs due to the expense of other household necessities. Moreover, they did not always share program leaders' understanding of this technology's effects or benefits as lifesaving malaria control tools. Turning global malaria control into a decentralized and at least partially privatized endeavor helped draw in resources for the cause, but it obscured the lessons scientists and health officials had learned over the 1980s and 1990s: ITNs were complicated interventions whose value—in terms of both utility and cost—were not obvious to intended users.

This chapter weaves together a portrait of ITNs' identity as global health commodities by tacking between "global" institutions and processes, such as Roll Back Malaria and its efforts to coordinate malaria aid, and on-the-ground efforts to implement ITNs in Africa. In doing so, it illuminates some of the ways international and national level public health activities influenced one another or, at times, did not. It surveys the activities of a range of organizations and experiences from around the continent, further emphasizing the heterogeneous and fractured nature of ITN distribution. The chapter ends by examining the cases of Tanzania and Zambia to illustrate how donors' ideal distribution strategies changed over the 2000s and to highlight the precariousness of control efforts based around global health commodities.

Creating a Global Market for ITNs

Roll Back Malaria catalyzed the mass dissemination of insecticide-treated nets in Africa, significantly expanding the scale of this intervention. It did this by making ITNs a cornerstone of its technical strategy and establishing itself as an obligatory passage point through which significant aid for malaria control flowed.[6] African countries' access to resources to mitigate malaria depended on their ability to carry out Roll Back Malaria's recommendations and on Roll Back Malaria's ability to attract those resources in the first place. Especially since donor agencies had shied away from malaria control in past decades, Roll Back Malaria leaders appealed to these agencies' interests and preferences, including their desire to link aid monies to measurable outcomes, such as the number of interventions distributed. The exigencies of attracting resources for global malaria control and demonstrating the impact of donor contributions reinforced the mass procurement and circulation of ITNs. In its position as a public-private partnership and self-described "brand and image" of global malaria control, Roll Back Malaria established a market for ITNs as global health commodities.[7]

Despite Roll Back Malaria leaders' substantial work to raise the international profile of malaria during the late 1990s and early 2000s, they struggled to attract the resources necessary to carry out malaria control activities during the partnership's early years. Therefore, Executive Director David Nabarro and other Roll Back Malaria officials initially spent a lot of time simply drumming up support for the new public-private partnership.[8] They tried to attract funding by emphasizing the link between malaria control and economic development, a tactic public health officials had used in the past.[9] The World Health Organization (WHO) director-general, Gro Harlem Brundtland sought to illustrate this link even more explicitly using data generated by the new WHO Commission on Macroeconomics and Health. The economist Jeffrey Sachs, the first chair of this commission, played a prominent role in promoting and publicizing the causal relationship between malaria and stymied economic development.[10] The United Nations (UN) also emphasized this link in 2000 by including malaria in the UN Millennium Development Goals (MDGs), which outlined a common agenda for reducing extreme poverty around the globe over the next fifteen years. Since these goals included reducing child mortality, improving maternal health, and "combat[ing] HIV/AIDS, malaria, and other diseases," donors could justify their contributions to international development through investments in malaria control interventions.[11] Such efforts to raise awareness and resources for malaria further consolidated the identity of ITNs as lifesaving goods that promoted economic development.

Roll Back Malaria officials relied primarily on development agencies for resources early on, so these groups' approaches to economic development significantly shaped how African governments implemented malaria control programs. The World Bank played a main role in defining this approach. By the late 1990s, bank economists, led by Chief Economist Joseph Stiglitz, pushed a modified orientation to development, often dubbed the "post-Washington consensus" or new development economics. They did so largely in response to the limited or, according to critics, detrimental effects of the bank's structural adjustment policies initiated the previous decade. This new orientation did not do away with market fundamentalism—the idea that the free market was the ideal mechanism for economic development and governance—which prevailed at the World Bank during the 1980s.[12] Rather, it acknowledged that in practice, the market contained imperfections, including those stemming from incomplete information or incomplete markets. In this framework states could, for example, help facilitate the circulation of health products by lowering taxes and tariffs on them, or fill in gaps in consumers' knowledge by running educational campaigns about the benefits of those products (both of which African countries did with ITNs). This orientation carved out a new complementary role for the state in public health, one in which the state worked to strengthen and make efficient markets of public health goods and services.[13]

This new development economics also maintained assumptions about actors and economies sometimes referred to as methodological individualism, which prevailed in the 1980s. Methodological individualism suggests that the economy is made up of individual agents all trying to maximize utility and value. This conception of the "homo economicus," or economic man, rests on the assumption that if people know about the benefits of a good or service, such as the lifesaving benefits of ITNs, they will purchase it, thereby strengthening that market. The World Bank, USAID, and other major development agencies perpetuated this methodological individualism in their approaches to disease control and poverty reduction. This informed their support for the mass dissemination of health commodities, such as ITNs, through the private and NGO sectors.

Recognizing that donors wanted to see the impact of their dollars quickly, Roll Back Malaria officials encouraged African country "clients" to triage malaria control activities strategically. Achieving quick wins by investing in those control activities "most likely to yield rapid and demonstrable success" was of the utmost importance to unlocking "additional internal and external resources for tackling malaria."[14] This recommendation encouraged countries to focus on scaling up ITNs, which were cheaper and easier to track than other parts of Roll Back Malaria's technical strategy, such as the early detection of epidemics or the prompt treatment of malaria. To demonstrate progress toward coverage goals, one could count how many nets had been distributed or how many people owned nets. It was possible to do this by tracking the activities of organizations involved in distributing nets, such as NGOs; one did not need to have a strong government health surveillance system in place. Moreover, some donors, such as USAID, initially did not even procure antimalarial drugs as part of its aid.[15] Many African countries continued to recommend ineffective drugs like chloroquine in malaria control policies, largely due to the high cost and lack of access to alternatives. During the early years of Roll Back Malaria, then, ITNs quickly came to play an outsized role in both African malaria control programs and in keeping the public-private partnership afloat.

Although ITNs had become high-profile public health tools, their tax identity initially impeded efforts to circulate them as such. Before Roll Back Malaria's launch, the market for bed nets in Africa was uneven and relatively small. Some textile companies and local tailors on the continent made these luxury items. However, with some exceptions, domestic supplies remained limited because potential consumers could not always afford bed nets at regular market prices and retailers did not always stock the item, possibly because of insufficient demand.[16] Most African bed net programs imported nets from Asia, particularly Thailand, and these were taxed as luxury goods. Meanwhile, the market for "public-health-grade" (as opposed to agricultural-grade) pyrethroids on the continent was so small as to be "virtually nonexistent," and many programs had to import insecticide from the United Kingdom.[17] Pyrethroids were often taxed as agricultural goods rather than public health goods, making them more expensive to import as well. Since most target consumers for ITNs tended to be poorer and ITNs were durable goods intended to last a few years, manufacturing of these products was a low-margin business.

Roll Back Malaria thus had to redefine and standardize ITNs as public health products to facilitate their widespread circulation. The partnership hoped this move would stimulate ITN production and ultimately reduce the cost of the intervention for both donors and African populations. Roll Back Malaria leaders called on African countries to reduce or waive taxes and tariffs on ITNs to make them cheaper to import. By offering subsidies to manufacturers to share the risk of developing products or promising to buy their ITNs, donor agencies encouraged these companies to scale up ITN production. The WHO Pesticide Evaluation Scheme (WHOPES) developed standards and recommendations for public-health-grade pyrethroids, regulating their circulation and use for ITNs. Roll Back Malaria and its various partners also sponsored trials of new products, such as bed nets with insecticide embedded in the fibers, helping to bring these onto the global health marketplace. Sumitomo Chemicals, Vestergaard-Frandsen, and SiamDutch Ltd., based in Japan, Denmark, and Thailand, respectively, took advantage of these new opportunities to become leading ITN manufacturers in the early 2000s. For Roll Back Malaria, managing global supply chains was part and parcel of addressing Africa's malaria crisis.

Even though Roll Back Malaria had successfully raised the profile of malaria control on the global stage, the partnership hit numerous setbacks that undermined ITN distribution. Little accountability existed among the partners, some of whom carried out activities ad hoc or lapsed on their funding commitments.[18] Competition with other health concerns, especially HIV/AIDS, for funding remained fierce. Many resources for Roll Back Malaria were also offered to demonstrate the viability of the public-private partnership model, rather than to support in-country control activities directly.[19] While the World Bank was a big-name sponsor, program officials noted that it "d[id] not operate in the world's most malarious counties," and most countries did not qualify for the bank's complex, "very difficult to access" loans for Roll Back Malaria activities.[20] African representatives complained about this slow trickle of funding, given how much pressure they faced to jump through Roll Back Malaria's hoops to access those resources.[21] And although the partnership's leaders promoted the idea that malaria-endemic countries had a say in Roll Back Malaria as full partners, countries could only apply for and access resources that donors wanted to provide. As more organizations joined the public-private partnership and set their own agendas and priorities, it seemed to some in the malaria control community that African "countries were ignored throughout all of that process."[22]

Therefore, while scientists and health officials realized that ITNs would not work as well in real-world conditions as in controlled experiments, the exigencies of attracting funding for malaria control ultimately drowned out calls for further investigation into how best to implement the intervention in specific African contexts. These needs also diverted attention away from calls to strengthen African countries' health sectors to sustain gains in malaria control, which Brundtland and Nabarro had articulated in their initial vision for Roll Back Malaria. Instead, Roll Back Malaria officials encouraged African countries to focus on demonstrating program success, primarily by reaching intervention coverage targets by 2005. To scale up ITNs quickly, these countries had to rely on various external partners, many of which had expertise in commodity procurement, marketing, and distribution rather than the technical aspects of malaria control or health systems. Those familiar with the complexities of malaria or implementing ITNs in Africa had limited ability to address those complexities, and the reification of these goods as global health commodities continued apace.

Scaling Up ITNs in Africa: Global Health Commodities on the Ground

Roll Back Malaria and its contributing partners may have agreed on the value of insecticide-treated nets, but that shared understanding of value did not always translate in national distribution efforts. Until about 2006–2007, at-risk populations who were supposed to take up the intervention did not do so in large numbers. This was particularly the case when it came to treating and re-treating nets with insecticide, which people were supposed to do to maintain the intervention's potency (at least until nets embedded with pyrethroids became more common after 2003). Since ITNs' ability to save lives depended heavily on high levels of use, the dismal coverage rates of both treated and untreated nets threatened the intervention's public health impact. Contributing to low uptake of the intervention was the fact that many countries initially used market-based distribution models that required people to buy bed nets and insecticide. While many scientists, health officials, and NGOs had already encountered these issues in trials and pilot projects from the 1990s, ITNs' momentum as global health commodities impeded efforts to fully address this obstacle.

As described in chapter 3, during the 1990s, groups working in a handful of African countries tried to distribute ITNs on a small scale using whatever resources they could assemble. In many cases, program leaders relied on NGOs and private voluntary organizations, such as the social marketing agency Population Services International (PSI), to help disseminate the intervention in cost-recovery schemes. Some governments and research agencies—for example, the Medical Research Council in The Gambia—offered free insecticide treatment on a limited basis to encourage people to take up the practice, but they did not have the funds to continue these efforts. They eventually introduced a fee to recover some of the costs of the insecticide, which led to massive reductions in treatment rates.[23] Despite lackluster results, charging people for nets and insecticide seemed to be the only economically feasible option for most countries, given the dearth of funding for malaria control. Furthermore, selling ITNs fitted structural adjustment reforms that aimed to decentralize and privatize African health sectors, as well rhetoric around community ownership and self-sufficiency popular in development circles at the time.

Roll Back Malaria largely maintained this model, where African countries would draw on whatever resources were available to scale up ITNs and pursue this activity in line with broader health sector reforms. While the partnership did not dictate how countries should disseminate the intervention, they strongly encouraged them to do so using social marketing. Again, earlier pilot projects did not suggest that this was an especially effective way to scale up ITNs and net retreatment, but with "little to no documented experiences to guide successful programme implementation," Roll Back Malaria officials sought a politically and economically viable approach.[24] The UK Department for International Development (DFID) and additional major donors to Roll Back Malaria supported social marketing and other market-based distribution methods in line with their neoliberal orientation toward health care provision. These donors hoped to foster the expansion of commercial markets for ITNs in Africa, where market forces—not governments or external aid agencies—would eventually sustain the distribution of this malaria intervention. For donors and Roll Back Malaria officials, social marketing would be a way to stimulate and create long-term demand (or a "culture") for ITNs in places where people were unfamiliar with the technology.[25]

Reliant on these donors for malaria control aid, many African countries embraced social marketing as well. PSI drew on substantial donor support to expand its role in distributing ITNs on the continent. Even though the social marketing agency's earlier bed net projects struggled to reach the very poor, donors and program officials hoped that greater investment in social marketing would help address outstanding issues and do so on a national scale. Increased funding, for example, could allow PSI to extend its behavior change communication campaigns into new areas or subsidize bed net and insecticide products to make them accessible to people who could not otherwise afford them. The ITN activities of PSI and other marketing agencies, described in a general sense here and elaborated in greater detail in chapter 5, offer a window into how these groups tried to sell Africans the value of this global health commodity.

Much of PSI's job involved creating demand for ITNs, which it did in various ways. Using marketing research surveys, the agency advertised the behavior of sleeping under and treating bed nets with insecticide to get people to adopt these practices—specifically in the cases of pregnant women and children under five. It circulated these messages via posters, radio spots, and other media outlets. PSI also created branded bed net and insecticide products, which they advertised and sold. As with its advertisements, the agency tailored its brands to different places. In Tanzania, for example, the agency sold Zuja Mbu (Stop the Mosquito) brand nets, while in Kenya, where fewer people speak Swahili, it sold Supanet nets. While this indicated some attention to different contexts, PSI's messaging was still rather generic and standardized. The language might differ, but the core points of the messaging remained the same. This approach matched the desires of global health programmers in being able to act efficiently, cost-effectively, and widely through cookie-cutter activities tailored to different places in shallow, trivial ways—a method well suited to the distribution of global health commodities.

In addition, PSI provided subsides for nets and insecticide to make them more affordable for poorer consumers. This included "cross-subsidies," which used profits from people who paid full price to subsidize nets for those unable to pay. Some program consultants worried that targeted subsidies might "crowd out" or "damage" fledgling markets if not managed correctly—for example, if people capable of paying full price somehow got access to a subsidized net intended for those unable to pay.[26] They suggested that PSI instead use subsidies for pump priming the market—basically using subsidies for a short period to increase people's exposure to ITNs, based on the idea that these users would then be willing to pay full price after experiencing the product's benefits. Since PSI and similar agencies could more easily track commodities and market inputs and outputs than they could malaria morbidity and mortality, they often knew more about the health of markets than about the health of people. Meanwhile, most African countries did not have the health surveillance infrastructure necessary to track morbidity and mortality data at a granular level, especially in rural areas that were hardest hit by malaria. As program leaders focused increasingly on how best to distribute ITNs quickly and within cost constraints, issues related to the contingencies and appropriateness of the intervention in achieving health outcomes fell by the wayside.

Other private voluntary organizations, such as USAID-supported Basic Support for Institutionalizing Child Survival and NetMark, used approaches that relied more strictly on the commercial sector to deliver ITNs to consumers. They discouraged subsidizing nets and insecticide from the outset since they believed that the people who benefited from these subsidies in practice were often those who could afford to pay the full market price. Instead, these organizations focused on building a self-sustaining commercial market targeting those who could pay in full first. NetMark, for example, initially directed its advertising at middle-class consumers who were more able to purchase nets but were not the primary targets of malaria control efforts.[27] Members of Roll Back Malaria's Resource Support Network for ITNs liked this approach for its cost-sharing potential, saying that "eventually all donor and NGO support should become unnecessary, allowing them to better focus on very poor populations who are not able to procure products through the commercial sector."[28] Such a strategy, of course, ignores the fact that the wealthiest populations are typically not the most at risk for malaria, and thus might not prioritize nets. Pregnant women and children who are the most at risk frequently do not have as much say over household purchases. Moreover, even people who have enough money might not have the funds to cover all their basic household needs along with an ITN. Roll Back Malaria and its partners had made building and manipulating markets core malaria control activities. In doing so, they took for granted that people would value ITNs.

Efforts to scale up ITNs using marketing techniques and price manipulation stalled in many countries during the early years of Roll Back Malaria. The behavior change communication activities of PSI and other agencies proved woefully ineffective. Early social marketing programs focused on simply raising awareness that malaria was a problem. This approach had its limits, as seen in Tanzania, where communities living near bed net re-dipping sites did not go to have their nets treated with insecticide even though they knew why and where to get treatment.[29] Noting the deficiencies of agencies' communication activities, Roll Back Malaria officials nonetheless felt that behavior change would emerge "with effective communication programmes, purposively directed at behavioural goals, and not directed just at awareness creation, or advocacy or public education."[30] In other words, they thought one just had to craft better messages to create enough demand to prop up bed net markets; the heavy reliance on behavior change communication to increase net coverage was not in question.

Manufacturers also tinkered with the technology to address one of the most difficult obstacles faced by national programs: getting people to treat and re-treat nets with insecticide. Until the mid-2000s people had to dip or wash their bed nets in insecticide, ideally every six months, to maintain their effectiveness in repelling and killing mosquitoes. Although this was essential to the intervention's ability to reduce malaria rates, especially in the context of low bed net coverage, many people did not treat their nets for various reasons. To get around this obstacle, manufacturers began making nets with insecticide embedded in the fibers, which maintained their potency longer through frequent washes. Vestergaard-Frandsen, Sumitomo Chemicals, and Siamdutch Ltd. all began making long-lasting insecticidal nets—PermaNet, Olyset, and Dawa Plus, respectively. Beginning in 2001, Vestergaard-Frandsen and Sumitomo Chemicals submitted their long-lasting nets for multi-village trials, which WHOPES officially approved in 2003.[31] As part of a corporate social responsibility initiative, Sumitomo Chemicals also transferred long-lasting insecticidal net manufacturing technology to A to Z Ltd. in Tanzania.[32] Although it took a few years to scale up this new technology, by 2006 long-lasting insecticidal nets constituted 70% of all nets distributed by African malaria control programs.[33]

Tinkering with nets and manipulating markets did not have a significant impact on ITN coverage during the early years of Roll Back Malaria. In 2003, just two years before African countries were supposed to achieve 60% coverage of at-risk groups, only about 15% of children under five in the African Region slept under untreated nets and about 2% slept under ITNs.[34] According to the WHO and United Nations Children's Fund (UNICEF) 2003 Africa Malaria Report, poverty posed one of the greatest barriers to scaling up the intervention. "The price of nets has fallen substantially as a result of greater demand, increased competition between producers, and reductions in taxes and tariffs and other obstacles to trade that many African countries instituted after the Abuja Summit," the authors explained. "Nevertheless, the commercial price of nets and insecticide . . . still puts this life-saving technology beyond the reach of the poorest income groups of the population."[35] Market forces alone, it seemed, could not fashion a working public health delivery system in the context of systemic poverty.

In response to these disappointing results, groups of malaria researchers, program managers, and other stakeholders engaged in an increasingly public debate about how best to distribute the intervention on the continent. An entomologist at the London School of Hygiene and Tropical Medicine (LSHTM), Chris Curtis, led the charge for free distribution through the public sector, comparing ITNs to vaccines: "We do not accept the view that scaling-up this method should be by making villagers pay for nets and insecticide, with subsidies limited so as not to discourage the private sector. We consider that [insecticide-treated nets] should be viewed as a public good, like vaccines, and should be provided via the public sector with generous assistance from donors."[36] In making this rhetorical link between nets and vaccines, supporters of free distribution highlighted the potential community-wide protections afforded by both interventions, at least when population coverage is high.[37] Jeffrey Sachs later joined the chorus supporting free distribution, lamenting with allies that "funds mobilised for malaria prevention and control are not used for saving lives, but are instead diverted to create new markets for bed nets that do not exist. This approach has compromised the effectiveness of malaria control efforts."[38] According to this group of critics, donors needed to ramp up funding for free ITNs to achieve an immediate health impact.

On the other side of this debate stood Christian Lengeler, Don de Savigny, Jo Lines, and some economists from the LSHTM. These researchers had helped develop Tanzania's ITN supply chain and voucher program with the Ministry of Health, domestic manufacturers (such as A to Z Ltd.), and other partners. They argued passionately for their specific private sector approach, which they felt would be more sustainable in the long run. In a response to Curtis and his colleagues, this group argued that supporters of free net distribution incorrectly assumed that one could not use markets to increase coverage, which overlooked evidence of progress in Tanzania.[39] With enough time, effort, and coordination, even those in poor, rural communities could come to value bed nets enough to pay something for them. Furthermore, the authors retorted, while advocates of free distribution cited China's and Vietnam's bed net programs—where the government provided insecticide treatment free of charge—as a model for Africa, those programs depended on people's buying bed nets from the private sector. Ordinary bed nets, they claimed, had always been private sector goods with no benefits to nonowners (in other words, with no "positive externalities"). Only when you added mosquito-killing insecticide did the object attain positive externalities and become a "public good" beneficial to nonusers as well. For them, it made more sense to subsidize the insecticide alone as the product that endowed the intervention with wider public benefit (as well as the product people were much less likely to purchase).[40] Most important, the group stressed that free distribution was simply not feasible with the present and foreseeable resources and would certainly cripple whatever commercial bed net market existed in Africa. "Curtis et al make bold statements about how the world 'should' be," Lines and his colleagues wrote, "but they do not address the question that confronts every programme manager: how best to use resources that are limited and that are not enough to do everything for everyone?"[41]

This debate endured for years as no side conceded. Lines, Lengeler, de Savigny, and others continued to support their painstakingly crafted supply chain, discussed later in the chapter, while Curtis and others rallied for increased resources to fully subsidize ITNs in Africa. One group believed that the necessary resources would not be there while the other argued that they *should* be there. "We went through five, six, seven, maybe ten years of flapping around in the international community with debates about what's the best thing to do," de Savigny recalled. "Do you do social marketing? Do you do vouchers? Do you do free net distribution, mass net distribution? And huge fights because there was no evidence one way or the other."[42] The ad hoc nature of global malaria control, combined with pressure to scale up ITNs quickly to reach coverage goals, almost certainly prolonged this lack of consensus.

Malaria program managers working in Africa responded to slow progress by experimenting with other distribution methods, including some that supplied free or highly subsidized nets, to increase ITN coverage with resources at hand. Some considered distributing the intervention as part of antenatal and public health services targeted to pregnant women and young children, such as national childhood immunization programs, to increase coverage in these high-risk groups.[43] Combining disease control technologies and maternal care services proved mutually beneficial for public health program managers. In Zambia a coalition of NGOs and development agencies funded a program that combined the distribution of ITNs, measles vaccination, vitamin A supplements, and mebendazole, which increased coverage of these interventions by 80% in the five target districts, according to a follow-up survey.[44] In Nigeria the Ministry of Health and partner agencies introduced ITNs into vaccination campaigns as "health incentives" in 2006. Even though many women seemed suspicious that polio vaccines were harmful, they took their children to get vaccinated in order to receive bed nets.[45] Such programs did not persist for very long in most places, often due to a lack of funding, though they certainly helped increase ITN use on the continent (to an average of 23% among children in surveyed countries in 2006).[46] In addition, these programs helped place ITNs into a broader meshwork of individualized global health goods woven, project by project, campaign by campaign across the continent.

Paying for Performance: ITN Distribution in an Age of Plenty

The massive increase in funding for malaria control in the mid-2000s eventually made moot many of the debates over how best to distribute nets in Africa. While the organizations most responsible for this increase broadened the possibilities for offering free insecticide-treated nets, as Curtis, Sachs, and others had called for, they constricted the possibilities for controlling malaria on the continent by only financing certain things. In particular, the politics, structure, and governance of these organizations privileged the rapid dissemination of commodities like ITNs through existing or temporary public health infrastructure, not through building up permanent health infrastructure.[47] The fact that these organizations emphasized paying for performance—or giving aid to places that demonstrated success in scaling up malaria control interventions and the capacity to measure that success—reinforced existing disparities between countries. This also created a feedback loop that encouraged the limited focus on procuring and disseminating ITNs.

The Global Fund to Fight AIDS, Tuberculosis and Malaria (hereafter the Global Fund) played by far the biggest role in financing malaria control efforts beginning in the mid-2000s, focusing on the mass procurement and distribution of ITNs and other commodities. The Global Fund's strategy of mass commodity procurement can be traced to the fund's origins during the AIDS pandemic. Public outcries over the astronomical price of antiretroviral drugs combined with gaps in funding for national AIDS programs during the 1990s spurred initial calls for a new financing mechanism at the beginning of the twenty-first century.[48] International health leaders proposed creating a commodity fund that would facilitate the bulk procurement of drugs, condoms, and HIV test kits, thereby lowering these products' price and transaction costs. They also felt that such a commodity fund could attract additional donors and grant funding for combating HIV/AIDS.[49] Representatives of the Joint UN Programme on HIV/AIDS (UNAIDS) stressed that a disease crisis of such great proportion in under-resourced areas required this kind of large-scale, immediate action. The logic of quick, massive commodity transfer shaped the development and activities of this new financing mechanism.

At around the same time that leaders of UNAIDS pushed for the new commodity fund, G8 countries recommitted themselves to fighting communicable diseases in low-income countries at their Okinawa Summit in 2000 in the name of health security and poverty reduction.[50] Prioritizing HIV/AIDS, malaria, and tuberculosis—the first two of which appeared explicitly in the MDGs—G8 leaders called for a new global movement to expand responses to communicable diseases that affected largely poor populations. The multi-institutional partnership that would be at the heart of the global movement would be based on "analysis of the ways in which poor people can be enabled to enjoy better health by increasing their demand for, and access to, useful goods and services," including by "marketing and subsidising the distribution of commodities such as insecticide-treated bed nets, condoms and even medicines through retail outlets."[51] Wealthy countries' plans to fight communicable disease and poverty in Africa and the global south centered on incorporating poor populations into the world capitalist economy. It was also premised on the idea that these groups were economically rational actors seeking to maximize utility—even if they had incomplete knowledge about and market access to health interventions.

International leaders proposed this "Global Health Fund" to correct the failures of public health commodity markets in Africa by providing commodities to people of few material means and to undeveloped markets in places where resources "can't be delivered by governments."[52] The fact that many African patients could not afford wildly expensive antiretroviral therapies, much less cheap nets and insecticide, challenged the idea that the free market alone would induce broad changes in consumption patterns and health behavior. Leaders of wealthy countries, however, felt that an infusion of money would be enough to fill gaps in markets, stimulate competition among manufacturers, and, eventually, bring down prices for poor consumers. Rapidly distributing lifesaving interventions—rather than bolstering the ability of at-risk populations to stave off disease or the ability of low-income countries to develop their own industries in health commodities—became a primary goal of global disease control.[53]

Participating country representatives formally approved the creation of a new global commodity fund to address tuberculosis and malaria along with HIV/AIDS at the 2001 G8 meeting in Genoa. Touted as "flexible" and "outcome focused," the Global Fund would operate outside of the UN system.[54] The US government found the global commodity fund particularly appealing. While it had not provided much funding at all for malaria control during the 1980s and 1990s, and was even slow to ramp up funding for Roll Back Malaria in the 2000s, it immediately partnered with the new Global Fund to become far and away its largest patron.[55] In addition, developers of the Global Fund adopted performance-based funding mechanisms—captured in the mantra, "Raise it, Spend it, Prove it"—to assure contributors that their donations were put to "effective" use.[56] The fund promised to satisfy donors' desire for accountability in their malaria control investments.

The Global Fund did not develop without reticence or resistance. Early in its inception, some government and development agency leaders expressed concerns about the new financing mechanism. The executive director of UNICEF, Carol Bellamy, thought that such a decentralized fund might "undermine our collective country level capacity building efforts" and focus too narrowly on purchasing essential supplies, which would "never be enough."[57] Even representatives at the WHO, an organization that once championed the building of basic primary health care systems, however, felt it was worth supporting this global commodity fund given the lack of other investment in malaria control: "WHO needs to advocate and support the global fund. [The Global Fund] is the major source of financing for the majority priority disease problems which WHO and countries have successfully advocated and mobilized for, set targets and . . . developed strategic operational plans and project proposals."[58] The precarious footing of Roll Back Malaria increased the appeal of this new extra-UN financing mechanism.

The heavy reliance of malaria control efforts on this commodity fund for resources, to the tune of 66% of all donor funding for malaria control by 2006, meant African health officials' possibilities for pursuing malaria control within broader health development projects shrank.[59] As one of the few effective malaria control commodities available during the early 2000s, and one of the only ones with its own global Roll Back Malaria goal, ITNs attracted a substantial number of newly available grants.[60] "Insecticide treated nets," in fact, appeared in 86.8% of Global Fund malaria proposals from the first four rounds of the organization's grant cycle.[61] The Global Fund had supported the procurement of 11.3 million treated nets by June 2006.[62] It has since remained the world's dominant buyer of ITNs—the most common malaria-specific commodity it procures.

Global Fund leaders' desire for experts in financial management and coordination often outweighed the desire for experts who were knowledgeable about the technical aspects of malaria. Decisions to fund malaria drugs contraindicated by the WHO due to high levels of resistance "seem puzzling," critics of the Global Fund decried, "until one realises that the [Global Fund's] Technical Review Panel is not actually a 'technical' review panel. The four malaria reviewers on the Technical Review Panel are selected by a points-based system, in which 'technical knowledge . . . and ability to judge whether proposals are . . . scientifically sound' count for only 22% of that decision. By contrast, 'familiarity with international processes and . . . partnerships' and 'familiarity with multisectoral approaches' count for twice as much (44%), even though it is hard to know what those criteria really mean [ellipses in the original]."[63] Creators and leaders of the Global Fund made sure to define the entity as simply a new financing mechanism, leaving technical review of the suitability of malaria interventions up to African countries and their external partners applying for grants.[64] Yet, by controlling the floodgates for malaria resources, the Global Fund exercised considerable influence on twenty-first-century disease control, sometimes in ways characterized as "medical malpractice."[65]

The Global Fund sought to include African officials' input by setting up Country Coordinating Mechanisms, a means by which in-country and external stakeholders put together grant proposals for the fund. These mechanisms were supposed to facilitate "co-investment" in disease control strategies, where public and private partners shared the burden of scaling up interventions.[66] The Global Fund did not, however, always coordinate funding through Country Coordinating Mechanisms in the first rounds of grant cycles, and instead gave grant money to NGOs. Roll Back Malaria officials recognized the threats that these mechanisms posed to country autonomy, noting in one 2005 report on performance-based funding that "partnerships are becoming another bureaucracy. They are duplicating existing structures and are absorbing financing and building their own capacity. Partnership mechanisms instead of supporting are taking over country ownership and leaderships."[67] Sending WHO or UNICEF experts, who were familiar with this bureaucracy, to assist in grant writing became a common solution to problems of African countries seeking money from the Global Fund.

Writing Global Fund grants became so critical to malaria control efforts that the Roll Back Malaria Secretariat, the US President's Malaria Initiative—a special bilateral aid initiative launched in 2005—and companies such as Exxon Mobil and Vestergaard-Frandsen (the biggest supplier of long-lasting insecticidal nets to the Global Fund since 2008) helped fund the grant preparation process in African countries.[68] African states essentially had to invest in the process of navigating external funding streams in order to acquire malaria control resources. Roll Back Malaria officials used the Global Fund proposal process to sell African health officials on Roll Back Malaria's technical strategy, noting that countries dedicated to coordinating malaria control efforts around the strategy had more successful grant proposals.[69] As a main pillar of Roll Back Malaria, which various public, private, and NGO partners could help procure and distribute, ITNs became a nearly ubiquitous component of successful malaria grant proposals. This financing process further reified ITNs as global health commodities applicable everywhere, regardless of social, political, economic, or ecological circumstances.

The problems of weak health systems and health data collection, of course, did not disappear with the influx of funding for malaria control. The Roll Back Malaria Working Group for Scaling-Up Insecticide-Treated Nets lamented the limited focus on commodities in 2005, claiming that while new investments by the Global Fund and others had made it easier for countries to procure malaria interventions, "relatively little investment has so far been made in the necessary health systems by which these goods can be effectively delivered to those most in need."[70] Lack of investment in monitoring and evaluation proved particularly crippling for countries seeking funding, since they had to demonstrate their progress in scaling up malaria control interventions to access Global Fund grants. "Most countries," a representative from the WHO-African region wrote, "have weak [monitoring and evaluation] systems which are not robust enough to be used to demonstrate any such performance."[71] New financing opportunities in global malaria control continued to privilege those national programs that enjoyed some degree of political stability and existing health and surveillance infrastructure. Moreover, these new financing opportunities reoriented African malaria control programs around the procurement and distribution of ITNs, including in places where changes in vector feeding and resting patterns reduced the intervention's effectiveness.[72]

Other organizations that contributed to the influx of aid for malaria control shared many qualities with the Global Fund, including its prioritization of accountability and investment in individualized technological solutions rather than health infrastructure or systems. The World Bank, which jumpstarted its support with its Booster Program for Malaria Control in 2005, operated in a similar pay-for-performance paradigm of aid provision. The bank agreed to provide roughly $500 million in additional funds over three years through the Booster Program to "reinvigorate" existing national programs that were struggling to procure and disseminate malaria control interventions. The bank emphasized accountability as a key aspect of the program, creating a results monitoring matrix "for laying out a more complete story on specific interventions such as the use of insecticide-treated bed nets, . . . from dollar per dollar investments to tangible on-the-ground results."[73] Such accountability practices, scholars have noted, privilege interventions most easily counted and measured rather than structural change.[74] World Bank representatives also claimed that the Booster Program would be "country-led" and that select interventions would be tailored to each country's, or "client's," specific needs. Their patron-client language glossed over the fact that African malaria control programmers had to tailor their requests to the desires and criteria of patrons who were able to provide resources. The countries that were most prepared and willing to scale up the sanctioned interventions received the most attention and support. And while the World Bank did not dictate how countries and organizations should distribute ITNs in Africa, it encouraged market-based distribution by funding organizations and programs that used this method, such as PSI and NetMark.

The Bill and Melinda Gates Foundation, led by the former Microsoft chief executive officer, Bill Gates, also promoted the pay-for-performance aid model. While the Gates Foundation did not focus as much on ITN programs specifically (concentrating instead on pharmaceutical, biomedical, and genomic research for malaria), it gave substantial amounts of money to the Global Fund. The performance-based funding mechanism and commodity focus of the Global Fund resonated with Gates's own emphasis on accountability, technological innovation, and empowerment through entrepreneurship—a libertarian approach to health and economic development that favors commodity-based solutions.[75] After it appeared that

Global Fund grants could help countries massively increase their coverage of malaria control interventions, the Gates Foundation set out to demonstrate that African countries could eliminate the disease with the right tools, logistical support, and commitment. As part of this endeavor, the foundation funded the Malaria Control and Elimination Partnership in Africa (MACEPA) and its activities in Zambia, discussed later in the chapter. The Gates Foundation has helped fund the supply of millions of ITNs through its efforts to demonstrate the viability of malaria elimination.

Although they contributed much less to the procurement of malaria control resources than these high-profile global health donors, humanitarian nonprofit organizations also perpetuated a narrow focus on distributing ITNs when they joined the malaria control movement in the mid-2000s. This group included a slew of new organizations dedicated to bed nets or malaria specifically, such as the Against Malaria Foundation (established in 2004), the Innovative Vector Control Consortium (2005), Malaria No More (2006), and Nothing But Nets (2006). Established religious charities, including Lutheran World Relief and Episcopal Relief and Development, also joined the effort, creating their own bed net programs that used "innovative and results-oriented approaches to saving lives."[76] And like Roll Back Malaria, the Gates Foundation, and others, these charities—some of which received funding from the Gates Foundation—advertised that their work saved and improved lives efficiently, under the assumption that someone spared bouts of malaria would increase their economic productivity.

As one of the "most efficient way[s] to save a life," ITNs, and specifically long-lasting insecticidal nets, became central to the activities of many malaria-focused nonprofits.[77] The nonprofit organization GiveWell, for example, ranked the Against Malaria Foundation highly and gave substantial money to this foundation, which focused solely on providing ITNs in malaria endemic areas. One of GiveWell's directors justified its support, saying that "giving out nets to prevent malaria has among the best evidence of any program that charity dollars can support worldwide, and more than 20 randomized controlled trials show it works . . . [giving out nets] is really cost-effective."[78] Humanitarian nonprofits mobilized the language of evidence-based public health to sell ITNs to philanthropic investors, NGOs, manufacturing partners, and publics in wealthy countries. This mirrored the concurrent popularity of randomized controlled trials in assessing development interventions, which were championed by the Nobel Prize–winning economists Abhijit Banerjee, Esther Duflo, and Michael Kremer, among others.[79] At the same time, ITNs came to be a source of value that nonprofit organizations could use to attract investments from GiveWell, the Gates Foundation, and other patrons to raise their own business profiles.

These malaria-focused nonprofits have procured tens of millions of ITNs for African countries over the past two decades. They typically arrange to distribute nets through international and local NGOs and private voluntary organizations, including the UN Foundation, Red Cross, and PSI, which are set up to do service delivery. On rarer occasions, nonprofit groups arrange to distribute nets through countries' national malaria control programs and government bodies. Nothing But Nets (now called United to Beat Malaria) also sends high-profile athletes and celebrities, such as the basketball player Stephen Curry and the television star Tom Cavanagh, on goodwill missions to hand out nets in African countries as publicity stunts meant to attract support, largely from audiences in wealthy countries. Bed net charities post pictures and videos of bed net distribution both to attract further donor support and, in some cases, verify that intended recipients are actually receiving the donated goods. In this way, photos and videos function as accountability mechanisms. By using these tactics, nonprofits have sought to convince everyone from individual to institutional donors that giving $10 for a long-lasting insecticidal net will translate directly into saving the life of an African child. These organizations too have helped circulate ITNs in the global health economy, transforming a once mundane tool into the center of a billion-dollar industry.[80]

Shifting Fortunes: Case Studies of ITN Distribution in Africa

Even though malaria control advocates and donors helped reify insecticide-treated nets as global health commodities that were circulated en masse to save lives in a cost-effective way, African governments and their partners did not all implement ITN programs in the same way. In fact, Roll Back Malaria officials looked to different countries' experiences to compile and adjust their program guidance. The National Malaria Control and Bed Net Programs of Tanzania and Zambia came to represent two different models for net distribution during the 2000s. Tanzanian officials focused on steadily building a domestic ITN supply chain and commercial markets— placing the burden of distribution on the private sector—while Zambian officials focused on the rapid scale-up of ITNs using significant external inputs. Roll Back Malaria officials and donors lauded each of these as an ideal in different periods, as the availability of resources for malaria control changed. A closer look at the development and fate of these two models illustrates the impact of sources and mechanisms of funding on the scale-up of ITNs in Africa.

Tanzania

Much like The Gambia, and later Kenya, Tanzania was an epicenter of ITN projects during the 1980s and 1990s. These included projects such as the Bagamoyo Bed Net Project, initiated in 1990, which aimed to develop a sustainable system for distributing and promoting ITNs using cost-recovery methods.[81] It also included KINET, a social marketing campaign with ITNs launched in two rural districts in 1996.[82] In all these projects, external research and development organizations worked closely with Tanzanian scientists and research institutions to investigate distribution mechanisms as well as the social, cultural, and economic factors that influenced people's decisions to adopt ITNs. While ITN research in Tanzania was not showcased in large-scale randomized controlled efficacy trials, it comprised a substantial base of knowledge about the uptake and use of this intervention in sub-Saharan Africa.

Building on this earlier work and experience, Tanzanian health officials and their expatriate partners moved quickly to formulate a national ITN distribution scheme following the launch of Roll Back Malaria—much more so than most other countries. The centerpiece of the National Insecticide Treated Nets Programme in Tanzania, also called NATNETS, was a national voucher scheme that provided pregnant women with subsidized vouchers that they could redeem at retail shops for low-cost ITN products. The scheme, based on a carefully crafted domestic supply chain, relied on and was meant to grow Tanzania's burgeoning bed net manufacturing industry. Ideally, donors and the Ministry of Health would subsidize vouchers that people exchanged for Tanzanian-made nets in commercial outlets, rather than procuring and distributing nets themselves. The scheme's architects embraced this approach in hopes of transferring the burden of ITN delivery completely to the private sector; they were pessimistic that the public health system could shoulder much of this burden over the long term.[83] At the dawn of the twenty-first century, after all, it was unclear whether and to what extent resources for malaria control would materialize. Research teams, moreover, had gained some traction in getting people to pay for nets and insecticide on a small scale in earlier pilot projects. Therefore, it seemed that forces of supply and demand could keep this public health intervention available in Tanzania for years to come.

Tanzanian health officials and their partners—including the WHO, UNICEF, the World Bank, and the Swiss Agency for Development and Cooperation—developed a proposal for a voucher scheme in 2000, though they did not have the resources to fully implement the scheme until the Global Fund came along. This promise of increased funding, however, did not provide an immediate fix. Richard Feachem, the first director of the Global Fund, was excited to award one of the fund's first-ever grants to support Tanzania's voucher program in 2002. "He kind of rushed the grant through" to be able to announce it at the upcoming Multilateral Initiative on Malaria conference, Don de Savigny remembered, "and then hit the wall because of the bureaucracy. . . . Suddenly this multimillion-dollar contract could not go to the [Tanzania] Ministry of Health because they had ceilings, fiscal space ceilings. That money had to go to the Ministry of Finance. And they had not got their ducks in a row. . . . The biggest, sort of, project the Ministry could receive in those days was thousands of dollars, not millions of dollars. And so there had to be a lot more things organized administratively for that to happen."[84] This issue of absorbing the influx of new global health funding available in the 2000s did not affect Tanzania alone. Many African health ministries, which transferred responsibility for health service financing to alternative institutions and adopted budget ceilings as part of structural adjustment reforms, had to adapt to these new financial circumstances as well.[85]

Roll Back Malaria officials presented Tanzania's voucher scheme as a model for scaling up ITNs in Africa during the first half of the 2000s, when the sustainability of donor support for malaria remained unclear. The Global Fund's promise of increased funding for malaria control commodities led Roll Back Malaria officials to think more seriously about strategies for making ITNs cheaper for vulnerable groups.[86] In a draft framework on ITN subsidies, Jenny Hill, Jayne Webster, and Eve Worrall touted voucher schemes, and Tanzania's National Voucher Scheme specifically, as a way to do so. "As programmes evolve and [insecticide-treated net] markets develop," they wrote, "it may be desirable to change from a subsidised goods approach to a voucher approach so that the public sector delivery system is alleviated of the burden of supply."[87] They acknowledged that such schemes were difficult to sustain without external support, were not well suited to places with weak commercial bed net sectors, and were "not ideal for very poor communities."[88] Program managers working with Roll Back Malaria nonetheless saw vouchers and commercial sector delivery as promising options since the public sector in many African countries appeared no closer to being able to support ITN supply and distribution themselves.

Ghana's Ministry of Health tried to initiate its own voucher program to help scale up nets in the country using Tanzania as a model. Drawing on support from various donors, Ghanaian health officials carried out voucher projects in the southern and central parts of the country beginning in 2003. While many African malaria control programs mixed and matched distribution and subsidy strategies in the early years of Roll Back Malaria, scraping together whatever resources external partners could provide, mixing in a voucher program did not work well. Different donors would only work in specific regions of the country, carrying out their own distribution strategies. As de Savigny explained, voucher schemes cannot effectively coexist with other approaches "because you need trust of the private sector to think that if you [a bed net manufacturer] make a net and put it there, someone's going to buy it with a voucher."[89] In the Volta Region, some health facilities continued to sell subsidized ITNs from a previous project after the voucher scheme began. In addition, commercial partners distributed many voucher-supported nets to health facilities, largely to the exclusion of commercial retailers. Due to low bed net stocks, retailers struggled to gain a foothold in the market— which is the ultimate aim of voucher schemes, since they are supposed to transfer the burden of distribution to the private sector.[90] As Ghana's experience makes clear, the Tanzanian state and its partners had to spend substantial time and effort building and coordinating ITN markets in the country; an uncoordinated provision of goods and logistical support, which is common in many global health projects, would not necessarily work.

One thing that separated Tanzania from Ghana, and indeed from many African countries trying to scale up ITNs, was the presence of a somewhat robust domestic bed net manufacturing industry. Sunflag, a textile company established by Satyadev Bhardwaj in Kenya during the 1930s, was the first company to manufacture bed nets in Tanzania in the 1990s. Then, around 1997, a group of researchers and members of PSI convinced Anuj Shah and Binesh Harria at A to Z Textiles Ltd. to enter the bed net market. They encouraged Shah and Harria to start making the green, rectangular nets that people in Tanzania seemed to prefer. Shah and Harria introduced their product at a meeting with the Chamber of Commerce, attracting the eyes and support of NGOs.[91] By 2004, two other textile companies in Tanzania had entered the bed net market as well, banking on purchases through the voucher scheme, though A to Z Ltd. remained the only company with the capacity to make long-lasting insecticidal nets.

Very quickly NATNETS and the program's key stakeholders, including Christian Lengeler, Don de Savigny, and Jo Lines, found themselves the opponents of those advocating for free bed net distribution. As noted earlier, advocates of free distribution argued for investing in public sector channels to help scale up ITNs in Africa, rather than assuming these channels were unable to do so.[92] Jeffrey Sachs and his allies even described Tanzania's approach as a failure, excoriating the idea of selling nets to people at risk for malaria.[93] Those supporting Tanzania's voucher scheme argued that the fluctuation and uncertainty of global funding for fully subsidized nets meant that African countries should work toward a distribution model that did not depend as much on continual donor funding.[94]

Tanzania experienced the risks of uncertain and volatile aid commitments firsthand after the 2005 World Economic Forum, where Sachs presented his message about free nets on a panel with the Tanzanian president Benjamin Mkapa, Bill Gates, and others. One member of the audience, the actress Sharon Stone, was so moved by the idea that ITNs could save thousands of children's lives that she agreed to donate $10,000 to Tanzania for the intervention. Rallying other members of the audience to add to her donation, she cried, "Just stand up. Just stand up. People are dying in his [Mkapa's] country today, and that is not okay with me!"[95] By the end of the forum, audience members had pledged to give Tanzania $1 million for free nets. However, not all those who pledged came through on their spur-of-the-moment commitment of funds. UNICEF agreed to make up the difference, giving about $860,000 of the $1 million so Tanzania's program officials could fulfill the purchase order they had already made.[96]

Many of those invested in NATNETS, including the architects of Tanzania's voucher scheme and domestic bed net manufacturers, were greatly dismayed by the prospect of this influx of free nets because it threatened Tanzania's supply chain. The managing director of Textile Manufacturers of Tanzania Ltd. (TNML), Anthony Haji, pleaded with the WHO director-general,

Jong-Wook Lee, to discourage this course of action. "It is . . . disheartening to learn that the Government of Tanzania together with some of its guiding partners are considering handing out more than 400,000 **free** nets to the Lindi and **Mtwara** regions to children under 5 years of age." Invoking Sharon Stone's outcry at the World Economic Forum, Haji continued, "The argument cited for the free nets is that these children need to be protected from malaria *today*. TNML fully understands the plight of these children and as a long-term investor in this country we are interested in the well-being of these children not only today, but yesterday, tomorrow and for many years to come (assuming we will still be around to produce and distribute ITNS)."[97] He felt that this massive donation might be more easily tailored to Tanzania's current approach—whereby donors covered the full cost of a voucher that people could trade for Tanzanian-made nets—rather than used to flood the market with free products. "In the long-run this is of course the only true and sustainable market from a private sector as well as public sector perspective."[98]

Haji's letter also shows that not all public-private partnerships were configured the same way. In one configuration, wealthy individuals and groups could give money to foreign ITN manufacturers and Tanzanian health officials would distribute the nets for free; in another configuration, Tanzanian officials could use external funds to buy nets directly from Tanzanian manufacturers via voucher subsidies. Interpreting the idea of public-private partnership in the latter sense, Haji complained, "Considering all the focus on our partnership as the way forward in public health in general, I find it exasperating that free distribution of nets is even considered as an option."[99] This predicament highlighted for Haji that partners did not "s[i]ng off the same hymn sheet."[100] Furthermore, his letter underscores an alternative value for ITNs—as a source of economic development for African countries—that became subsumed by the object's value as a cost-effective, lifesaving good for foreign donors looking to disseminate nets en masse.[101]

In practice, Tanzania's National Voucher Scheme increased ITN coverage across the country only very gradually. According to one survey, the proportion of households in the country owning at least one ITN increased to just 29% by 2007, though just as many households owned at least one untreated bed net.[102] Furthermore, only 25.7% of children under five and 23.2% of pregnant women used ITNs—rates well below the 60% Abuja Declaration target.[103] Those living in urban areas and wealthy households were more likely to own and use bed nets. As in many previous cost-recovery projects, the cost of nets and insecticide proved a barrier to ownership and use, especially among the poorest populations. Researchers also linked low usage rates to some people's lack of knowledge about the connection between malaria and mosquitoes and low levels of promotion in certain districts, mainly those in the western part of the country far from former bed net project sites and Tanzania's main urban centers.[104] While the voucher scheme did help increase ITN access in outlying, rural areas of the country, it by no means solved the problems with delivering the intervention in Tanzania, which had been identified as far back as the mid-1990s.[105]

Tanzania's National Malaria Control Programme continued to operate the voucher scheme even after newly available resources from the Global Fund allowed African countries to conduct free mass ITN distribution campaigns beginning in the mid-2000s. Roll Back Malaria officials referred to free mass distribution activities as "catch-up campaigns," intended to increase coverage rapidly either as a stimulant in areas where communities had not adopted ITNs widely, or as an effort to replace people's old, worn-out nets. Defenders of Tanzania's voucher scheme tried to emphasize the importance of "keep-up," or continuous distribution, alongside catch-up campaigns since the latter could not effectively accommodate new pregnancies and births.[106] As more donors, NGOs, and humanitarian organizations joined Roll Back Malaria, however, and latched on to ITNs in particular, more and more African countries switched to relying heavily on free mass distribution campaigns. Tanzania's slow and steady coverage growth suddenly paled in comparison to the very high coverage rates of neighbors who blanketed regions with free nets. The country even organized a free distribution campaign in 2008 in response to findings of low ITN coverage. By the end of the decade, Tanzania no longer represented an ideal model for ITN distribution or malaria control development in Africa.

Tanzania's voucher scheme finally ended in 2014, under pressure to meet donors' pay-for-performance criteria. Tanzanian health officials adopted the free mass campaign model in its wake. In addition, in 2015 the Tanzanian government changed the classification of ITNs from zero-rated goods (that are not subject to value-added taxes due to, for example, their societal importance) to exempt supply goods (that are subject to these taxes). The government did so as part of a broader effort to significantly reduce domestic tax-exempt items and increase state revenue.[107] This change meant that domestic bed net manufacturers had to raise the price of their products to continue making a profit, putting them at a severe disadvantage in competing for Global Fund tenders. Most companies cannot compete for such tenders anyway because they do not make WHOPES-approved long-lasting insecticidal nets, which donors seek out.[108] Following the subsequent influx of cheap bed nets from Asia, A to Z Ltd. and Sunflag laid off thousands of workers amid stagnant bed net sales.[109] The twenty-first-century global health economy, built on the global, cost-efficient circulation of health commodities, may have facilitated the saving of lives, but it has severely damaged African-led efforts toward sustainable health and economic development.

Zambia

Zambia emerged as a demonstration ground for a very different approach to scaling up ITNs in Africa during the 2000s. Specifically, the country used substantial external resources to increase ITN coverage very quickly. This approach grew out of the pressure felt by malaria control advocates to demonstrate success to donors and secure additional resources for malaria control in Africa. It also depended heavily on the mass of new funding available in the mid-2000s, which did not exist when Tanzanian officials first developed their national voucher scheme. Members of Zambia's National Malaria Control Centre and their partners provided proof of concept that achieving high coverage of ITNs and other Roll Back Malaria interventions could reduce malaria rates to levels approaching elimination (bringing the incidence of indigenous cases of malaria in an area down to zero). At the same time, the country's experience illustrates the risks posed by fluctuating donor inputs, both to the distribution strategy and the health of populations in malaria-endemic areas.

During the first years of Roll Back Malaria, Zambia's National Malaria Control Programme adopted social marketing as its strategy for distributing ITNs, which Roll Back Malaria partners favored at the time. This strategy built on Zambia's bed net activities from the 1990s, in which NGOs and development agencies supported small-scale, cost-recovery projects at the district or community level. Although leaders of the national program recognized that entomologists working with the WHO recommended "targeted vector control" for malaria control programs, they also "recognize[d] that in the current resource-poor environment in Zambia," measures like indoor residual spraying, larvaciding, and eliminating breeding sites were "not cost-effective . . . for the public sector."[110] Thus, Zambian officials maintained the focus on insecticide-treated materials in the country's malaria prevention and vector control activities.

Zambia also benefited from private sector involvement in funding malaria control. In 2000 the Konkola Copper Mines helped fund malaria control in the country's Copperbelt Province, specifically the districts of Chingola and Chililabombwe. Using indoor residual DDT (dichlorodiphenyltrichloroethane) spraying—the vector control method of choice in Zambia's mining regions during the 1970s and early 1980s—this effort proved successful in reducing malaria cases in the two districts. Malaria control officials cited this as a good example of "how collaboration between the private and public sector can benefit the community and business," an example followed most notably by ExxonMobil in West and Central Africa.[111] Zambia drew on further investments from industry to expand this effort beyond Chingola and Chililabombwe and demonstrate the viability of a multipronged approach that included indoor residual spraying, which the WHO had discouraged for use in Africa during the 1990s and early 2000s on the basis that countries would not have the capacity to carry out spraying effectively and sustainably.

Investment and success in malaria control continued to advance hand in hand in Zambia. In 2003 the Roll Back Malaria Secretariat selected the country for a consultative exercise in which WHO/Roll Back Malaria experts would help Zambia's Ministry of Health negotiate a support package from outside partners and donors. The Roll Back Malaria director, Fatoumata Nafo-Traoré, acknowledged Zambia as "one of the countries in Africa with the greatest potential, and readiness" to achieve Roll Back Malaria targets since the country had adopted many of the global partnership's recommendations— including reducing taxes and tariffs on ITN commodities, mobilizing additional resources for malaria control, creating "effective partnership mechanisms," and completing a situation analysis and strategic plan.[112] Zambia had also proved its success in obtaining malaria control funding from the newly created Global Fund—one of only seven African countries to do so in Round 1 of the organization's grant cycle.[113] The World Bank committed roughly $20 million to Zambia through its Malaria Booster Program, citing the country's efforts to reform and decentralize the health sector during the late 1990s and the government's commitment to Roll Back Malaria as evidence of aid worthiness. External funding for malaria control in Zambia grew from about

$9 million in 2003 to nearly $40 million in 2008.[114] In an era of performance-based funding, the country emerged as a frontrunner in the scramble for malaria control resources.

It was Zambia's connection to the Gates Foundation, however, that catalyzed its emergence as a demonstration ground for a new way of scaling up malaria control. In 2004 the Gates Foundation funded a program within the Seattle-based, nonprofit Program for Appropriate Technology in Health (PATH) called the Malaria Control and Elimination Partnership in Africa. According to Rick Steketee, a former longtime member and science director of MACEPA, this program was created to sustain the pursuit of malaria control at a time when endemic countries in Africa struggled to scale up interventions. "Roll Back Malaria was risking not having a success to build on, that no country was actually demonstrating the successful scale up of all of the recommended interventions," he told me. "And the donors were sitting on the sidelines, not necessarily diving in. . . . Our notion was that the world needed some successes, and that success at a national level would be required, not at a sub-national level."[115] Drawing on help from Roll Back Malaria, in particular from James Banda—a member of the Roll Back Malaria Secretariat and contact person for Zambia's malaria control program—MACEPA's leaders chose the country as the testing ground for a new strategy they called "Scale-Up For Impact."

Scale-Up For Impact was supposed to provide an alternative to fractured, slow-moving social marketing projects and to achieve high coverage of "evidence-based" interventions. ITNs, indoor residual spraying, and case management "were proven effective interventions, they had a lot of science and clinical trials behind them, but nobody was taking them to high coverage in populations," Steketee recalled. "But the idea was if you look at bed nets as a vaccine that saves lives, vaccines save lives on the basis of coverage. So it was all about coverage."[116] MACEPA coordinated support among the donor community for the new strategy, tapping into supporters' interest in demonstrating and tracking the impact of their investments.[117] MACEPA provided a competing model for scaling up ITNs, which officials summarized as "sound policies attracting partners and growing resources."[118]

Zambia turned out to be a place well suited to MACEPA's demonstration project, due in part to the country's political stability, along with the Ministry of Health's commitment to and history of collaboration with external partners on malaria control. MACEPA consultants helped plan the National

Malaria Control Strategy for 2006–2010 and mobilize resources and logistical support to scale up the interventions. A portion of donor funds went toward strengthening the routine health management information systems needed to track and illustrate the success of the Scale-Up For Impact strategy—a chief aim of the endeavor.

Beginning with Luapula and Western Provinces, Zambian malaria control officials and their partners at MACEPA began scaling up ITNs around the country in earnest around 2006. They tapped into and expanded existing networks of district health workers, NGOs, and community-based organizations to distribute these commodities, even using infrastructure originally dedicated to HIV/AIDS activities. Piggybacking off other health services as well, Zambia's National Malaria Control Centre and its partners subsidized ITN distribution through antenatal clinics and routine child health services, including childhood vaccination campaigns. They complemented these efforts with mass bed net distribution campaigns in rural, hard-to-reach areas, distributing over 3.5 million ITNs in 2006 and 2007 and reaching over 60% coverage with the intervention in the northeastern and western parts of the country by 2008.[119] The National Malaria Control Centre maintained commercial ITN distribution in urban areas, where they focused instead on scaling up indoor residual spraying.

As health officials carried out these activities, health and demographic surveys showed a 29% decline in child mortality from 2001 to 2007. The surveys also showed a 69% reduction in severe anemia prevalence among children under five from 2006 to 2008, and a 54% reduction in malaria disease incidence among children in this age group over the same two-year period.[120] While these nationally aggregated statistics do not capture heterogeneity of health impact in places such as the marshlands of Nchelenge District, they seemed to substantiate Scale-Up For Impact as a success.[121] Thus, MACEPA representatives mobilized such data to argue, "Zambia is demonstrating that it can be done!"[122]

Bill Gates lauded efforts in Zambia to scale up malaria control tools at the 2007 Malaria Forum meeting in Seattle, saying, "Zambia is an inspiring example of a nationally-coordinated effort. Three million long-lasting insecticide-treated bednets are being distributed there this year, and the country is close to reaching its national target of 80 percent of households with at least one net—up from 20 percent two years ago."[123] Even more amazing, Gates claimed, representatives from other African countries were now discussing with malaria funders how they could follow Zambia's model of scaling up interventions nationally. In convincing potential donors of Zambia's success as a model, Gates and MACEPA officials made little of the fact that Zambia is not representative of numerous other endemic countries in Africa, where political and economic circumstances continually limit, threaten, and undermine malaria control activities. By portraying malaria control as a technical problem that could be solved by getting commodities and interventions into people's hands and homes, they collapsed the variability that separated Zambia from other countries.

Moreover, this picture of the rapid distribution of ITNs was not quite as rosy as Gates portrayed it. Not everyone who owned an ITN actually used it. "The intervention was assumed to be a known and popular one," researchers reported, which underpinned assumptions that "fast and near universal uptake would arise because (1) the intervention is known to work (protect from malaria); . . . ITNs are relatively cheap/free; . . . [and] ITNs are easy to use."[124] However, the presumed lifesaving value of ITNs did not determine people's responses to the object. Survey data showed that of those families in Luangwa District who received ITNs in a 2008 mass distribution campaign, just over half of recipient children slept under one during the period of data collection.[125] Even with substantial communication campaigns in the district and high levels of awareness of the intervention's benefits for malaria control, many people did not hang up the nets they received, making the device wholly ineffective as a health intervention. Just because ITNs circulated widely in the larger economy of global health goods based on evidence of their biomedical efficacy, it did not mean that they retained this efficacy as they entered African households.

While Zambia had enjoyed significant external support for its malaria control activities during the mid-2000s, this support fluctuated; this fluctuation had disruptive and detrimental effects. External support for malaria control and ITNs in Zambia slowed dramatically in 2009, following the mismanagement, or disappearance, of a grant of 7 million Swedish krona (about $700,000) to Zambia's Ministry of Health. Other donors followed Sweden's lead in withdrawing funding for Zambia's Ministry of Health shortly thereafter. The European Union and Global Fund began funneling support through UN agencies rather than through the ministry, making it more difficult for Zambian health officials to direct money to its priority areas.[126] Because Zambia was highly dependent on external donors to support the country's health sector, health service delivery—including antenatal services that incorporated bed net distribution—suffered. Malaria illness and mortality rates increased with the disruption in funding and service provision in the eastern part of the country, which is more rural and where malaria transmission is more intense.[127] Rates of insecticide resistance also increased, as they have across the continent. In its 2011–2015 Strategic Plan, Zambia's National Malaria Control Centre recognized the need to build up human resource capacity and health infrastructure to help prevent shocks caused by fluctuating funding. At the same time, it recommitted the country to addressing these gaps in the health system by pursuing universal coverage of malaria control interventions such as ITNs.[128] Just as Zambia demonstrated the viability of Scale-Up For Impact as an ideal approach in an age of high donor interest and investment in malaria control—and especially in funding cost-effective health commodities—so too did the country demonstrate the precariousness of malaria control under these new conditions.

As ITNs became increasingly central to malaria control in Africa over the 2000s, they became crystallized as global health commodities—standardized items exchanged in a marketplace of global health goods for their value in the cost-effective saving of lives. Those who participated in rolling back malaria in Africa bolstered and operationalized this identity in pursuit of their own interests, which often included reducing malaria for economic and humanitarian reasons, but also frequently for securing financial resources. In the process, these groups divorced ITNs from the conditions of their use, which could vary widely across a single country, much less an entire continent. They also separated the technology from the reality that children in resource-poor settings die from multiple, interrelated causes "and it is hard to identify which health interventions spared a life."[129] The idea that ITNs could save children's lives regardless of social, cultural, economic, or ecological context initially empowered marketing models based on demand creation, which rested on assumptions that consumers would invest in the intervention for its biomedical value. Such deterministic conceptions led policy makers, program managers, patrons, and manufacturers to tinker with ITN markets, supply chains, and technology to address the problems with scaling up nets, overlooking many of the barriers scientists encountered in getting people to use nets as intended or in pursuing malaria control in Africa in other ways.

Furthermore, prevailing beliefs among the development community that poor populations were comprised of autonomous, rational economic actors seeking to optimize utility and value reinforced support for demand creation strategies. For the development community, providing African populations the means to access a tool of survival, whether through commercial markets, highly subsidized channels, or charitable donations, meant giving poor people the means to pull themselves out of poverty and suffering. Such conceptions of ITNs as a technological fix for economic development diverted attention away from the politics of dependence and power inequities in global health, which was in fact reinforced in the rise of ITNs.

5

The Domestic Technology

Making Healthy Homes in Kenya

Today, many Kenyans acquire insecticide-treated nets through various inroads of global health and development, whether public health campaigns, nongovernmental organization (NGO)-led projects, or antenatal clinics. This is particularly true in the country's more impoverished, rural areas where people cannot afford to buy nets—certainly not at full price. Those with means and access, however, can also pick up an ITN at Tuskys, Nakumatt, and other large retail stores for about US$10. Despite the object's status as a main pillar of global malaria control, you will not find it stocked alongside other health products in the medicine aisle. More likely, you will have to go to the home goods section, where you will find an array of other mosquito nets of different shapes, sizes, colors, and fabrics. This arrangement of consumer goods is a reminder that this object never lost its identity as a household item, even as its importance to public health changed during the late twentieth century. In fact, by transforming and disseminating ITNs as a public health intervention, scientists and health officials spurred the technology's widespread domestication across Kenya, sub-Saharan Africa, and the global south more broadly.

Bed nets are among many objects that illustrate how the enterprise of global health and development has increasingly extended into the personal lives and homes of the world's poor populations. Personal water filters, clean cookstoves, and, in some places, ready-to-use therapeutic food have proliferated via foreign and philanthropic aid, becoming fixtures of daily domesticity in Africa and elsewhere in the global south.[1] The neoliberal character of global health and development has played a role in this process, promoting decentralized, market-based governance, greater participation from private and nongovernmental sectors, and individualized commodity interventions. High-level political and economic policies alone, however, do not explain how, why, or when Kenyans adopted ITNs. For years after the launch of Roll Back Malaria, many people did not purchase or internalize the value of nets as lifesaving goods as policy makers and programmers had hoped. Getting intended users to do so required substantial work and depended heavily on Kenyan scientists, health officials, health workers, and other bed net users—much as it did during bed net trials in Siaya and Kilifi. Kenyans did not simply take up the intervention according to theories and plans developed outside the continent; rather, they engaged in acts of "constitutive appropriation," refashioning and integrating bed nets into their sociocultural world to serve their own diverse ends.[2] Sometimes these ends included protecting their households from malarious mosquitoes, but at other times they did not.

This chapter continues to explore the history of ITNs' implementation as evidence-based global health technologies by examining how and why Kenyans domesticated these objects following the launch of Roll Back Malaria.[3] As on the continent more broadly, ITN distribution in Kenya was a patchwork effort, financed and operated through a variety of organizations. These groups not only worked to help Kenya reach Roll Back Malaria coverage goals but also produced knowledge about ITN distribution and use among poor rural populations. Kenyans' patterns of consumption ultimately informed global ITN policies, specifically recommendations to disseminate nets through free mass distribution campaigns. Focusing on the experiences of residents of the former province of Nyanza—a region with some of the highest malaria rates in the country and the site of numerous ITN projects—the chapter highlights the influence of Africans' interests and practices on the enterprise of global health.[4]

Understanding the Early Life of Bed Nets in Kenya

To understand the uptake of insecticide-treated nets in Kenya—or anywhere targeted for the intervention—one needs to understand the longer history of this technology in the region. While ITNs were new technologies in Kenya in the late twentieth century, ordinary (untreated) bed nets were not. Residents' prior experiences with bed nets informed their responses to the new intervention as it became an increasingly prominent part of public health activities. Although not universally shared across the continent, these experiences draw attention to the ways that class, gender, and colonial relations shaped people's interactions with this household item.

Before the advent of Roll Back Malaria, many understood bed nets as luxury goods, associating them with urban settings, *wazungu* (white people or foreigners), civil servants, educated people, and wealthy inhabitants. Indeed, bed nets initially proliferated across the global south through European efforts to survive and colonize the tropics. While European colonists and other *wazungu* may have used nets to protect themselves from disease-transmitting insects, not everyone shared this idea of the object's utility. One woman I interviewed, for example, originally thought that white people used nets to protect their skin from unsightly mosquito bites.[5] Unsurprisingly, then, many people I talked to in rural areas of Nyanza said they had not used bed nets until relatively recently. Earlier, if they did try to keep pesky mosquitoes at bay, they often did so by burning cow dung, *mieny* (*Lantana camara* plant), or smoke-emitting mosquito coils. Many nights, they did not do anything but swat mosquitoes "left, right, and center."

Gendered colonial labor and migration patterns meant that those who were most familiar with bed nets in this early period were men. Gem resident John Obonga recalled buying a bed net in Nairobi during the late 1950s for 120 shillings, "a very expensive price in those days." Even in Nairobi, he said, bed nets "were not common in the past. They were only common among soldiers who came back from the war in 1945 and among police."[6] Tom Ochangwa, on the other hand, said he first encountered bed nets in his school during the early 1970s. "You know I went to a boarding school. These other schools had no such [mosquito nets] because they were not boarding schools. . . . Even the homes here [Gucha] . . . had no mosquito nets."[7] Bed nets were not always connected to education or high-status positions. One *mzee* (elder) said he first used a bed net while working on a tea plantation in Kericho, harvesting one of the colony's most important exports.[8] Nor did people describe using bed nets for malaria prevention specifically, more often saying they used them to block mosquitoes. This fitted common ideas that mosquitoes were not a source or the sole source of malaria.[9]

Women who used bed nets in this earlier period often did so because of their relations with fathers, husbands, or other male kin. Anastasia Akinyi grew up with bed nets as a child because her father received some when he was stationed in Bombo, Uganda, as part of the British colonial army. "We used to have the nets, right from the time we were children," she told me. "During the time when we came back to Kenya the authority was in the hands of the white men. So all those working, and more especially those working with the government, all those who had big jobs and had money would buy the nets."[10] These relations were not always kin based. Victoria Okech, a Catholic woman living in Asembo, said she first obtained a net in the mid-1970s through a Dutch missionary named Father John. Father John worked at the Pandpier Catholic Centre in Kisumu, where Victoria and her grandmother lived at the time, selling bed nets and training people to sew them. Happy to give up the pungent smell of burning cow dung, Victoria embraced mosquito nets.[11]

While some Nyanza residents had used bed nets before these became an important public health intervention, they did not consider bed nets goods for the "common *wananchi*," for ordinary people.[12] "Before the government came in," one man summed up, bed nets "were being brought in and assimilated to the communities by those people who had been in towns who have known [malaria] mostly in the lake region, where they understand that the mosquito is very, very great. So they brought these things. They had even been buying them themselves. . . . A majority in the community cannot afford to buy, so they went through the ministry of health."[13] When researchers and malaria control programmers began to introduce ITNs into rural communities, they did so in this wider context of associations and meanings—a context in which poor women and children typically did not use these luxury items, and bed nets were not necessarily linked to malaria. To scale up ITNs in the country, they had to redefine bed nets not only as public health tools, but as interventions intended especially for society's most vulnerable populations.

Marketing ITNs under Roll Back Malaria

Roll Back Malaria prompted the Kenyan government to massively scale up insecticide-treated nets across the country. Working with various donors, NGOs, and other external agencies, Kenya's Division of Malaria Control aimed to reach 60% coverage of both pregnant women and children under five (designated as "vulnerable groups") with the intervention by 2005. While this effort significantly expanded previous ITN activities undertaken during the 1990s, it maintained certain elements of those activities, including selling the intervention to at-risk populations. This reflected the government's continued reliance on outside organizations to finance and operate

ITN programs and donors' desires to sustain this malaria control intervention by creating a consumer market for it. These political and economic realities, layered on top of the history of bed nets in Kenya, proved to be major obstacles to the dissemination of ITNs during the first half of the 2000s.

Population Services International (PSI) took the lead in scaling up ITNs during the first years of the Roll Back Malaria program in Kenya, as it did in many African countries. Drawing substantial funding from the UK Department for International Development (DFID), PSI launched a national social marketing scheme in partnership with Kenya's Ministry of Health and Division of Malaria Control in 2002. The agency aimed to distribute 2.4 million nets to vulnerable groups through supermarkets, small shops, and other retail outlets to "stimulate the emergence of a net culture" and, eventually, a self-sustaining commercial market for the intervention.[14] In theory, this would save donors and the Kenyan government from having to continually procure ITNs or build new public health infrastructure.

PSI undertook a variety of activities, including tracking bed net ownership and use. It dedicated much of its work, however, to behavior change communication, designing both unbranded and branded advertising campaigns to sell people on the idea of using ITNs. In both types of campaigns, the agency disseminated messages through conventional mass media channels such as print, radio, and television. The agency predominantly conducted this messaging in Swahili or English, Kenya's two official languages, to reach as wide a swath of the population as possible. Of course, these materials were not accessible to everyone, especially where people had low levels of education and predominantly spoke in a different mother tongue. PSI tried to address this gap by using mobile cinema units in impoverished rural areas, where many people were illiterate and did not own televisions. It also organized community drama performances, educational rallies at market centers, and other "culturally appropriate" venues to advertise the intervention.[15] This work did not rely on the expertise of those intimately familiar with the technical complexities of malaria control, but rather on those with skill in marketing, business, and behavioral social sciences, along with Kenyan interlocuters.

Much of PSI's early messaging, moreover, focused on simply raising awareness that ITNs were malaria control tools, with the assumption that this information would lead Kenyans to purchase and use the intervention. PSI's unbranded, generic bed net advertising portrayed malaria as a silent killer that took the lives of young and unborn children. These ads then told people to sleep under an ITN. Meant to be generalizable, this advertising appeared in many other African countries during the early 2000s. Certainly in Kenya, this generic messaging appeared to have little effect on people's uptake of or desire for ITNs. According to one of PSI's surveys, many Kenyans found this kind of "shock and fear campaign" too negative and disjointed.[16] Early ads did not make the link between sleeping under a net and preventing malaria explicit. For example, one poster pictured a smiling girl running in between two child silhouettes, and read, "Malaria huua watoto 36,000 walio chini ya miaka mitano kila mwaka. Hakikisha wako analala ndani ya neti ilyotibiwa kila siku" (Malaria kills 36,000 children under five years every year. Make sure yours are sleeping inside a treated net every night).[17] This did not make the value or function of ITNs clear to those who did not understand mosquitoes as the cause of malaria, even if they considered malaria an important health problem. And even those who linked malaria to mosquitoes did not always perceive malaria symptoms—which overlap with symptoms of many other illnesses and might correspond to various local illness categories—as a sign of this vector-borne disease.[18] The revelation that people unfamiliar with bed nets did not immediately understand the tool's medical importance was not new, of course. Scientists working in Kenya and across the continent encountered—and worked hard to overcome—this obstacle in bed net trials during the 1980s and 1990s. It therefore seems that consideration of this epistemic divide did not travel well from controlled experiments to mass marketing campaigns.

PSI was more successful in raising awareness through its branded campaign. This campaign drew on a common idea in social marketing that one can sell a product-based behavior (such as sleeping under a bed net or using a condom during sex) by branding and selling the associated product. In 2001 the agency relaunched its "Supanet" brand bed net, which it had first developed for its social marketing pilot project in Kilifi the year before.[19] PSI also introduced a new insecticide sachet, "Power Tab," complete with its own superhero champion, Mr. Power Tab.[20] This branding played up the connotations of strength, power, and protection and helped distinguish these products from ordinary bed nets associated mainly with comfort. PSI bundled Supanet and Power Tab in a home treatment kit to encourage people to re-treat their nets with insecticide, an ongoing challenge that had persisted since the first pilot projects with ITNs.

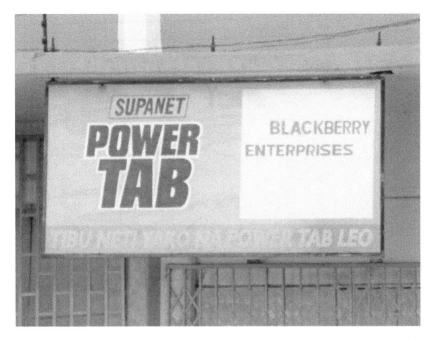

Storefront in Kisumu town, Kenya, 2015 (Translation: "Treat your net with Power Tab today"), photo by author

PSI disseminated its branded products through existing private sector channels. In urban areas, it sold the products through a network of distributors, who then sold them to wholesalers and retailers. In rural areas lacking big commercial outlets, PSI sold its products through small kiosks and shops. The agency agreed to paint shop exteriors with social marketing messages at no charge if shop owners agreed to sell Supanet and Power Tab products alongside their other goods, not all of which were medicine- or health related.[21] Some of these faded exteriors remain today, literally paling in comparison to newer, brightly colored messages of recent bed net distribution efforts. Over time, ITNs became integrated into Kenya's built environment, not only inside homes, hotels, and shops but also onto the structures peppering cities, townships, and the countryside.

PSI priced its products differently in different parts of the country, recognizing that people living in urban centers like Nairobi tended to have more disposable income than populations in rural areas. During the first couple of

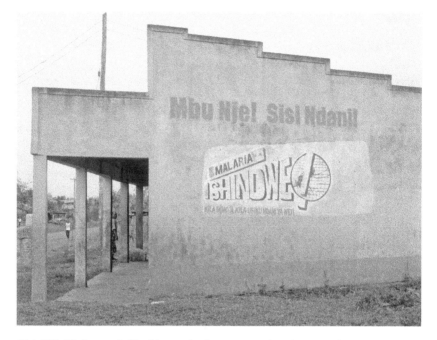

Old PSI-Ministry of Health marketing messaging in Luanda, Kenya, 2015 (Translation: "Down with malaria"), photo by author

years of the program, PSI sold nets for 350 Kenyan shillings (KSh) (roughly US$5) in urban areas and between 100 and 140 KSh (roughly US$1–2) in rural areas.[22] The agency planned to use money made from unsubsidized sales to subsidize nets in rural areas. To prevent "leakage," where people buy cheaper subsidized nets in rural areas and sell them in urban areas for a profit, PSI introduced differently colored and shaped nets for each region: green, rectangular nets in rural areas and white or blue conical nets in urban areas.[23] They used this approach in other countries as well, tinkering with both the market mechanisms and the bed nets themselves to try to scale up the malaria control intervention.[24]

Kenyan malaria control officials and their PSI partners struggled to increase ITN coverage among target groups during the early years of the program. For example, PSI dedicated a lot of its resources and energy to selling nets in urban areas such as Nairobi, where malaria transmission was extremely low.[25] The agency did this in part because more robust communication and marketing infrastructure, as well as in-country bed net suppliers, existed

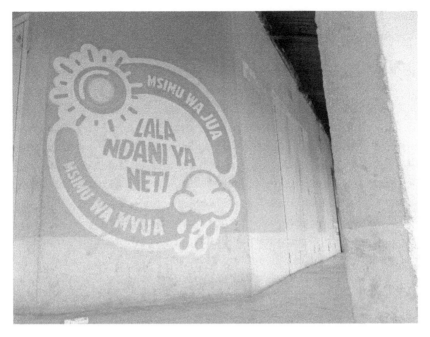

More recent PSI-Ministry of Health marketing messaging in Nyawara, Kenya, 2015 (Translation: "Sleep inside a net during the dry season and rainy season"), photo by author

in these areas. PSI representatives also felt that sales in urban markets could eventually support higher subsidies in fledgling rural ones, justifying their continued investment in the former.[26] While this may have made some sense from a business perspective, it left behind many of those who lived in higher-risk rural areas.

The price of the product also presented a major obstacle to distributing ITNs on a national scale, though this was not unexpected. While PSI's social marketing program had "created considerable demand for [insecticide-treated nets]," Kenyan officials reported at an Eastern Africa Roll Back Malaria Network meeting, "even at subsidised prices they remain unaffordable to certain sectors of society," such as rural populations and poor urban inhabitants.[27] Although 100 KSh was a relatively a cheap price for a net, around half of the country's rural households made less than 1,500 KSh per month, most of which they spent on food.[28] Kenya's 2003 Demographic and Health Survey highlighted this disparity, showing that bed net ownership among people in the highest wealth quintile dwarfed that among people in the lowest wealth quintile by over 20%.[29]

Gender also intersected with geographies of poverty and disease in ways that did not align with initial plans for ITN distribution. Male heads of households often controlled finances, and they did not always prioritize nets for their wives and children.[30] In Nyanza, male household heads also frequently migrated to urban areas or large commercial farms for work, leaving wives and children to care for rural homesteads.[31] In many cases, then, women had to buy bed nets for themselves and their children on their own with monthly income that fluctuated based on season, familial obligations, and a host of other factors. These dynamics complicated efforts to increase ITN coverage among pregnant women and young children.

Furthermore, Kenyan consumers did not always do what program leaders wanted or expected them to do. Many people refused to buy or accept white nets, feeling that these looked like ghosts or burial shrouds, thus associating them with death. Some thought that sleeping under a white rectangular net was like sleeping in a coffin.[32] Rectangular nets were commonly sold in rural areas. While this boxy design provided more ventilation, some complained that the net did not always offer adequate coverage. "It is the adults who use the nets instead of the children because children sleep in groups on a mat," one woman explained. It is "difficult to hang a net over a large mat. If you hang it on the roof, the net is too short, if you fix it on the wall it covers only half of the mat . . . and there is no large net to cover a large mat with a group of children" [ellipsis in the original].[33] Since families could not always afford multiple nets, this mismatch between bed net design and rural domestic spaces hindered public health aims.

Behavior change activities in rural areas also sputtered, in part because many people did not see ITNs as having "any health benefits."[34] Older ideas about bed nets as items for comfort endured. PSI also did not have enough boots on the ground to fully monitor leakage, which allowed some people to resell bed nets or insecticide informally for a profit. Drasilia, a woman I interviewed in Asembo, speculated that the nets being distributed in Kenya in 2015 lacked insecticide sachets because program officials discovered that women were selling the "insecticide soaps."[35] While that is not the reason nets no longer come packaged with sachets of insecticide—which is now embedded in net fibers—her speculation suggests a more dynamic circulation of ITN products in Kenya than quantitative surveys reveal.

Indeed, the challenge of getting people to treat their nets with insecticide remained a major problem. The cost of buying new insecticide discouraged some from treating or re-treating their nets. Many people also cited confusion about where to buy more insecticide and mentioned the burden of preparing and washing nets in insecticide as reasons to forgo the practice. This burden almost always fell to women and girls who tended to domestic chores, among many other tasks. Although PSI's bundled ITN package contained instructions, some did not feel they had enough information about how the insecticide worked to use the chemical on their nets. This information was important because if the nets were not dried properly, the insecticide provoked rashes, itchy skin, and coughing fits. "Whenever you would use the nets after washing from the insecticide, it had some pungent smell that would choke someone. You will feel like the chest is locking, and you would be forced to open the window," one man recalled. "It even prevented many people from going to buy the insecticide."[36] Household income significantly shaped ITN coverage in Kenya, but price was not the only barrier to use.

PSI and Kenyan health officials modified their strategies in response to people's ideas and practices with ITNs. For example, they changed where they sold the product. At the international level, the Roll Back Malaria Secretariat organized meetings and facilitated communication among African health officials from around the continent to share insights and experiences with scaling up ITNs. According to Kiambo Njagi, a longtime member of Kenya's National Malaria Control Programme, this kind of information sharing was useful in negotiating with external partners. "One time we went for a bed net meeting with my boss in Zambia," he said,

> and we shared experience with a number of countries within the region and we realized our idea of selling bed nets through kiosks is not working. And therefore, when we came back, we decided to sit with PSI, modify their policy. . . . . And we told them, "look . . . you can continue with the kiosks, but besides these kiosks, let's involve health workers more. . . . because we're targeting under [five] and pregnant women—let's put these nets at maternal-child health [centers], so that as these women come for their antenatal clinics, as these people bring their children for immunization, the nurse who is a health worker can also promote nets. And those who want to buy can buy. Okay?"[37]

PSI started distributing ITNs through antenatal clinics in partnership with the Ministry of Health and Division of Malaria Control, beginning on the Kenyan coast in 2004 and expanding to all fifty-one malaria-prone districts the following year.[38] This system continued to operate with user fees, as clinic staff were supposed to buy ITN products from PSI for 30 KSh and then sell them to pregnant women for 50 KSh. The 20 KSh profit could then be put toward more nets, infrastructural improvements, and recurrent facility costs.[39] This method of distribution, along with lower prices, stimulated increased ITN coverage of children under five from roughly 4% in 2001 to about 24% in 2005.[40] "The uptake really picked up," Njagi recalled, "because now it is the health worker, not a villager talking to another villager, . . . trained to convince a villager the health benefits of this commodity."[41] While this solved some problems, Kenyan officials noted that "there [wa]s still a proportion of populations that cannot access these nets," and felt "a need for more subsidized nets."[42] Meanwhile, some dispensary workers admitted, they might sell nets to people outside target groups to be able to recover the costs of the intervention and sustain health services. They also did so to address complaints and alleviate suspicions that nets were reserved for certain groups.[43] Manipulating elements like product, price, place, and promotion—the "4 P's" of social marketing—to reach target consumers with ITNs was an incredibly complex task and did not always work out as predicted.

PSI also revamped its behavior change messaging to more clearly articulate the connection between sleeping under ITNs, blocking mosquitoes, and reducing malaria. Around 2004 the organization developed the new campaign slogan for Kenyan markets, "Malaria Ishindwe!" (Down with malaria!), based on surveys showing that preachers often used "ishindwe" in calls to combat demonic forces.[44] In 2009, after the Global Fund and other donors had begun financing free mass distribution, PSI launched another advertising campaign that coupled Malaria Ishindwe! with the slogan, "Mbu nje! Sisi ndani!" (Mosquitoes outside! Us inside!).[45] PSI included icons that paired mosquitoes in a red "no" symbol with the phrases, "Komesha Malaria, Okoa Maisha" (Banish malaria, Save lives) to further emphasize the connection between mosquitoes, malaria, and survival.

PSI also found in its surveys that social norms heavily shaped bed net use. If people thought everyone else was using this product, then they would be more likely to use it as well. This was reflected in some of PSI's posters, which featured people tying up, tucking in, or sleeping under bed nets, and paired these with messages about the tool's benefits for one's community and family. One poster, for example, showed some women hanging up a net as onlookers clapped, reading, "Hata tuwe na shughuli nyingi namna gani, lazima tu-hakikishe kuwa, kila mmoja, kila usiku, analala ndani ya neti, ili kujenga jamii bila Malaria" (No matter how busy we are, we must make sure that everyone, every night, sleeps inside a net to create a society without Malaria).[46] PSI also used images of health workers using nets, emphasizing the health function of the intervention. This messaging encouraged personal and community-led vigilance about domestic malaria control practices. Especially after 2007, when the World Health Organization (WHO) recommended that African countries pursue universal coverage with ITNs (net use among all household members in at-risk areas, regardless of age or gender), PSI also included more images of men in its ads, though women continued to feature prominently in caretaker roles.[47]

Scaling Up Nets, Producing Knowledge

While PSI conducted insecticide-treated net activities across the country, other organizations also operated smaller-scale, time-limited proj-ects with the intervention. Consequently, ITNs covered the country unevenly, concentrated not only among better-off segments of society but also among poor communities enrolled in research studies.[48] Many of these projects, in fact, sought to intervene in debates about the viability of providing free nets to address low coverage rates among poor populations. Through this frac-tured effort, Kenya became an important terrain on which academics, health practitioners, and development agencies produced knowledge about African poverty, ITNs, and health.

Several NGOs distributed nets in pilot programs aimed at improving maternal and child health. For example, in 2003 the economists Jessica Co-hen and Pascaline Dupas created the NGO named TAMTAM Africa, Inc. (To-gether Against Malaria, Tuafue Afya Na Maisha), which provided free nets and HIV/AIDS counseling at government clinics in Busia, in western Kenya.[49] As the two received pushback on the approach, the project morphed into a research study on how pricing affected bed net uptake and use among poor populations. "I was trying to get money for the NGO," Dupas recalled,

and I was at a meeting in Silicon Valley. . . . People were like, "What? You give bed nets for free? That's crazy. People aren't going to use them. Don't you know that people don't use things that they get for free?" . . . I realized that there was such a very strong sense that free stuff was bad because it was not used. And somehow it didn't click with me because, you know, with marketing in the US or Europe, you get free samples all the time for stuff. So I was like, "Why are people saying it's okay to get free stuff if you're rich, but if you're poor, it's not?"[50]

These "Silicon Valley types" argued that consumers would not value something they did not pay for and that, for consumers, low prices indicated low product quality. They also argued that consumers who spent a lot of money on a product would feel bad not putting it to use—a sunk-cost effect. Dupas and her colleagues sought to test these ideas, generated from western economic and marketing frameworks, by tracking how many of the women they served used and "valued" ITNs after receiving one for free.[51] They did so as part of a growing movement in development economics to apply experimental frameworks, such as randomized trials, to test development interventions.[52]

Although initially they were not confident that free distribution was the best way to encourage bed net use, according to Dupas, their research seemed to validate the approach nonetheless. An initial survey showed that roughly 85% of women who received free nets were sleeping under the nets one year later.[53] Some of those who did not use nets were planning to give them to their children when they went off to boarding school; others were waiting to build a separate cooking hut unconnected to their sleeping spaces so the net would be not be stained with smoke or catch fire.[54] This initial work spawned further studies of bed net use and pricing in Kenya and beyond.[55] While some people took the results to heart, the findings did not have a major effect on actual programming. "It seemed like there were always people on both sides of the debate within any organization. And [the study] just created some evidence base the pro-distribution camp could use" and "tip the debate in some cases."[56] But neither public health practitioners nor journalists cited the research much in discussions about free distribution and pricing. "It's a problem that, essentially, economists write in a way that is totally unappealing to anyone else," Dupas laughed, "no one reads an economics journal."[57] The lack of consensus on how best to distribute ITNs opened opportunities for inquiry and intervention during the early 2000s, but momentum, funding priorities, and budgetary constraints ultimately favored fee-based methods.

Scientists from the Kenya Medical Research Institute and US Centers for Disease Control and Prevention (KEMRI-CDC) also distributed ITNs, specifically to the population in Asembo and Gem as part of their randomized controlled trial during the late 1990s. They continued to distribute free nets there in 2001 and 2002 as they tracked the long-term effects of the intervention on malaria rates. Local *nyamrerwa* (community health workers) working for the CDC continued to carry out educational and surveillance activities, as researchers organized mass dipping campaigns in schools and village centers. Monitoring adherence to the intervention alongside child mortality and malaria morbidity, KEMRI-CDC scientists also generated data supporting the argument for free distribution to at-risk populations. "Results demonstrate that populations who are given bednets for free and who do not have a history of bednet use can learn to appreciate the benefits of bednets and improve adherence after initial acceptance," they argued.[58] They noted, however, that some residents of the study area still did not use the intervention as scientists and health officials had intended, even under controlled research conditions. "It appeared clearly that bednet as an obvious 'thing' is well perceived," one analyst wrote, "but not the 'plus' conferred by the insecticide itself, and this could explain the low rate of retreatment often observed everywhere."[59] Again, price was a common barrier to use but not the only one. The way that people understood ITNs and the technology's function also mattered.

In Nyawara, a sublocation in Gem, residents gained some exposure to ITNs through KEMRI-CDC's bed net trial. More than through the medical research partnership, however, people remembered receiving nets through the "Millennium" or *"maendeleo* (development) people." The "Millennium people" were representatives of the Millennium Villages Project, a rural development project and brainchild of the economist Jeffrey Sachs. Sachs, who became director of the UN Millennium Project and Columbia University's Earth Institute in 2002, intended the project to serve as a laboratory for development in Africa. In 2004 he and his colleagues established the first Millennium Development Village in Bar Sauri, Kenya. They quickly expanded the project to cover ten other sublocations in the "Sauri cluster," including Nyawara. As Sachs described in *The End of Poverty*, after an initial site visit, project representatives felt that they "would be able to put some of the ideas to work in Sauri and help the international community learn from the experience in Sauri for the benefit of villages in other parts of Africa and beyond."[60] An outspoken advocate for free ITN distribution, Sachs and his colleagues included free nets in this development project.

The NGO running the Millennium Villages Project there began distributing free long-lasting insecticidal nets on a two-year cycle around 2005. At that time, malaria prevalence totaled about 55.8% among children under five and 49% among the cluster's entire population. Unsurprisingly, malaria prevalence was highest among the poorest residents.[61] The NGO trained *nyamrerwa* to teach residents how to use the nets and to survey the region for proper bed net use. It is difficult to determine how successful free ITNs were in stimulating economic development, as the project promised. However, the introduction of the intervention correlated with declining malaria prevalence in Sauri, a greater decrease than that measured among those living outside of the cluster.[62] Like many other projects in Kenya, the Millennium Villages Project saturated the region with nets and knowledge related to malaria, health, and development but did not repeat this elsewhere in the country.

Modeling Free ITN Distribution

Kenya's Division of Malaria Control and Ministry of Health coordinated with these various partners to socially market ITNs and support small-scale projects examining the viability of free distribution. It also got more directly involved in efforts to test distribution strategies, seeking to weigh in on issues of equity, access, and effectiveness of malaria control. In 2001 Sam Ochola, the head of Kenya's Division of Malaria Control, worked with researchers at the University of Oxford on a twelve-week pilot study of free distribution.[63] Health workers at antenatal clinics in thirty-five districts gave pregnant women free nets and insecticide procured by the United Nations Children's Fund (UNICEF). Surveys from Makueni and Kwale indicated that most recipients were using the nets after one year.[64] Analysts stressed that the project "clearly showed that large scale distribution of [mosquito nets] and insecticide is feasible *with currently existing systems*," such as antenatal clinics, making cost-recovery projects unnecessary.[65] "These findings show that free bednets are valued and used by recipients. This important information needs to be included in the debate on how to scale-up bednet delivery to vulnerable groups."[66]

As members of KEMRI-CDC also recognized, though, distributing free products did not automatically solve all the problems plaguing distribution efforts. Miscommunication about the intended use of ITNs remained an issue. Sometimes health facility staff did not provide information to recipients about how to treat the net with insecticide, an activity that was critical to the public health function of the technology, though it was not intuitive.[67] Some pregnant women, moreover, did not use nets while pregnant under the impression that nets were only for the baby. Ensuring that only vulnerable groups like pregnant women and young children used the free nets also proved difficult. At least one person in the survey area had sold off their free net to someone else.[68] Overall, in fact, about 20% of the 70,000 bed nets UNICEF procured ended up with nontarget groups. This included men, who, as the main income generators in their families, used bed nets to keep themselves healthy so they could work.[69] Giving out free ITNs to mothers did not entirely remake the household relations and economic realities shaping net use.

Kenyan malaria control officials and their partners did not have the resources to continue distributing free ITNs, though they did continue to sell the product at antenatal clinics for about 50 shillings to target pregnant women and children. In some cases, women even traveled longer distances to attend maternal and child health clinics that offered cheap ITNs.[70] Antenatal clinics and hospitals served as a common entry point for many women in rural areas to learn about bed nets and malaria. Still, women had to assimilate this knowledge into existing routines and sleeping habits, a process that was not intuitive, especially in situations where new mothers and children did not sleep together. "When I . . . went to clinic and was given only one net for the first born," one woman told me,

> I would at times place the baby on the seat to sleep, and didn't put a net because I was using the net in the bedroom. So the child ends up being sick. Now I wonder. When I go to hospital, I tell them "the child is now again sick and suffering from malaria." Then they told me "it's because you placed the child on the seat. The mosquito doesn't know that the child normally sleeps under a mosquito net. So any time your child is sleeping, you need to put the child under the net." So when I did that, my third born has never gotten sick or suffered malaria.[71]

Of course, getting to a clinic in the first place was difficult at times and not simply due to issues of geographic access. "During those times, there was a problem with HIV tests," one woman recalled. "As long as you're an expectant mother you had to go through it. There was a lot of stigma, so many women did not go to hospital. They preferred to give birth with the midwives. But I was lucky. I went to hospital and got a net."[72] Domesticating ITNs as health technologies in Kenya was a complicated process shaped by the social world of illness, gendered work and care, and rural poverty.

Kenya benefited from the tremendous influx of external funding for malaria control in the mid-2000s. Drawing on technical assistance from the

WHO and funding from DFID, Kenyan health officials successfully applied for a Global Fund grant in 2004 to procure and distribute roughly 3.4 million long-lasting insecticidal nets for children under five.[73] This grant represented the largest successful award for the free distribution of long-lasting nets in Africa to that point, and international malaria control advisers praised Kenya as a model fundraiser that other countries could learn from.[74]

Kenyan malaria control officials planned to distribute the long-lasting nets in western Kenya through an integrated measles vaccination campaign in July 2006. As with antenatal clinics, they used vaccination campaigns to deliver nets to target groups, in this case children under five. Kenyan officials looked to other African countries that had already tried this strategy for guidance. "It all started in Zambia, and we saw that it could be done," Njagi recalled. "When Togo was distributing bed nets, their first mass nets [campaign] in 2004, we sent a delegate from Kenya to go and observe how the logistics of such massive nets is conducted. Luckily, I was among the delegates."[75] Health officials from different African countries shared their experiences with each other, building up a base of programming knowledge for colleagues who were also under intense pressure to scale up ITNs to meet Roll Back Malaria goals.

It turned out that Kenya's Division of Malaria Control did not have to wait until July to test out its integrated bed net-vaccination campaign. In September 2005, health officials detected the beginning of a measles outbreak among Somali immigrants in Nairobi, .[76] District health officials initiated vaccination activities early in sixteen districts in central Kenya, taking the opportunity to try integrating measles vaccination and bed net distribution before the planned campaign. During this test run they found that many distribution centers had run out of nets by the second day, in part because mothers had figured out ways to obtain extra nets.[77] Officials adjusted their distribution techniques for the July campaign, marking children's fingers with a pen to indicate who had already received nets and vaccinations. District officials and their partners were fairly successful using this distribution method, increasing ITN ownership among Kenyan households with children under five to about 67%.[78]

Again, free ITN distribution helped address the problem of financial access but did not always lead directly to use. The Division of Malaria Control found that even though 67% of households received a free net, only about 42% had an ITN hanging in their house and only about 52% of children were reported to have slept under one the previous night.[79] In more extreme cases, recipients rejected free nets altogether. In Kilifi, some people spread rumors that the nets were "talking" to their users, giving children fevers and inducing hallucinations.[80] They believed that they would have to sacrifice their first- and last-born children in exchange for the net helping their other children. Focus group interviews revealed that some were suspicious of outsiders coming in to give goods away unconditionally and that there must have been an ulterior nefarious motive at play, especially since the nets seemed to be reserved for certain groups. They did not, as many economists claimed, take the free status of bed nets as a mark of poor physical quality, but responded in ways that reflected a longer history of exploitation. Health workers, chiefs, and other local authorities tried to assuage people's fears and explain the benefits of sleeping under ITNs, since it seemed that this information did not reach all recipients during the campaign.[81]

Indeed, a more common scenario encountered by health officials was that people simply did not share officials' ideas about the primary value and purpose of nets. "Some people who were given those [nets] who do not know why they were given, they tore the nets to cover their gardens," one woman explained.[82] People in Kenya and across the continent redefined ITN commodities in many other ways as well, incorporating these malleable meshworks into their particular domestic spaces and household economies.[83] What was one person's mosquito barrier and malaria prevention measure was another person's fishing net, curtain, chicken coop, blanket, wedding veil, outdoor latrine covering, rope, or bag for carrying produce. Many also appropriated ITNs in different ways over time, using them as protection from insect pests until they became too worn and torn to keep away hungry mosquitoes. These acts of everyday innovation came into the spotlight as academics, health officials, and journalists sought to characterize the nature and extent of the alternative use or "misuse" of subsidized global health goods.[84]

During the first mass distribution campaigns, moreover, some did not understand why they were suddenly receiving nets. "Did you ever get a free net?" I asked one *mzee*. "Yes," he said, though he did not remember the exact year. "A majority of people," he continued, "don't have these memories of when the nets were distributed for free because, one, if you're in class, you know you are learning for a given goal. The nets are being given, but [recipients] do not know the next motive or the next goal, or the future goal for why

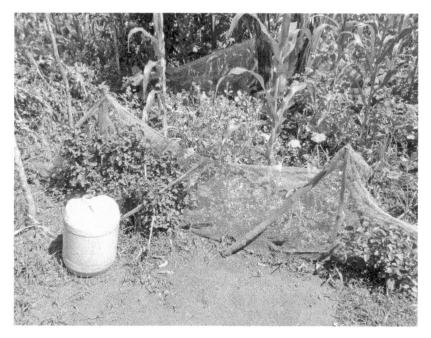

Bed net used to fence in a vegetable garden in Kisii, Kenya, 2015, photo by author

the nets are being distributed. So that is why a majority of people do not keep track of what year they received the nets."[85]

This is not to say that those distributing ITNs in Kenya's first mass campaign completely neglected to provide information; only that the provision and reception of information seemed to be uneven. Gender shaped this dissemination of knowledge, with women often receiving more ITN messaging through health projects and antenatal clinics as primary caretakers of children and (in the case of pregnant women) as part of a vulnerable group themselves.[86]

Making Global Health Practice in Kenya: Evidence for Free Mass Campaigns

Despite Kenya-based researchers' and health officials' calls for fully subsidized insecticide-treated net distribution, the money and resources did not exist to support this on a large scale during the first half of the 2000s, and debates over how best to disseminate the intervention persisted. In this context, Kenyan researchers from the KEMRI-Wellcome Trust partnership in Nairobi monitored and compared results of ITN uptake across four sentinel sites in the country. They overlaid this study on continuing efforts by PSI and the Kenyan government to distribute ITNs through various means, including social marketing campaigns and, in 2006, free distribution. Ultimately, they produced statistical research findings showing that fully subsidized net distribution was the most equitable distribution method and had the greatest public health impact—findings that the WHO used to sanction free distribution as the best way to scale up the intervention in Africa. In this way, Kenyan researchers and residents who took up and used ITNs shaped the continent-wide domestication of this technology.

Even though it took many years for Roll Back Malaria leaders to decide on an effective strategy for scaling up ITNs in Africa quickly, researchers sought to answer this question early on. Under the direction of Bob Snow and the KEMRI-Wellcome Trust partnership, researchers in Kenya used mapping, database, and survey technology to assess access to malaria interventions and health facilities in the country. One of these scientists, Abdisalan Noor, came to KEMRI in 2000 specifically to work on this project using his background in engineering, global information systems, and geospatial analysis. "Bed nets were working. We knew that from the clinical trials," Noor remembered. "There were a number of suggested approaches to scaling up, . . . but nobody knew what was really the best way to scale up and the best way to sustain, and whether they were equitable, [and] cost-effective. And the second thing that was unknown is, how did communities, when they got the intervention, how did they actually accept it? How did they use it? How often did they use it? What was the impact on parasitemia? What was the impact on mortality in an operational setting?"[87] Working in conjunction with the Ministry of Health, Snow, Noor, and the rest of the team set out to answer these questions for Kenya.

KEMRI-Wellcome Trust's research was heavily shaped by past and concurrent ITN distribution in Kenya. "We decided with Bob we were going to set up seventy-two villages across four different ecologies: . . . eighteen in Bondo, eighteen in Kwale, eighteen in Makueni, and eighteen in Kisii/Gucha," Noor recalled.

And we followed them up, I think, once after every high transmission season over a period of five years. And did lots of household type surveys, including birth histories, to document deaths, and all that. And the beauty of that study—and this was largely coincidental—was we started when the main intervention for scaling up bed nets was through social marketing, largely conducted by PSI. Then, subsequent to that bed nets [were introduced] through clinics to under-fives and pregnant women. Then free mass campaign. . . . And we were able to look at how access to bed nets varied in terms of just general coverage but also in terms of equity and impact.[88]

Researchers' selection of study sites reflected prevailing understandings of and approaches to malaria in twenty-first-century Africa. The four districts selected for the study mapped onto the varying epidemiological conditions in Kenya, from intense perennial transmission in the lakeside region of Bondo to the acutely seasonal, low transmission of Makueni in the semi-arid south. Researchers also noted that a majority of households in the rural areas of these districts lived on less than US$1 per day, well below the poverty line.[89] Thus, communities involved in the study came to function as important proxies for populations most at risk for malaria, not only in Kenya but in sub-Saharan Africa more generally. Randomly choosing approximately 2,687 homesteads from across the four districts, researchers created a longitudinal cohort of children under five that they surveyed in 2004–2005 and 2006–2007.[90]

Researchers tracked both ITN and malaria disease indicators over the two-year study, stratifying study populations in the four sentinel sites by wealth quintile (from most poor to least poor). They accumulated evidence that fee-based distribution discouraged or disadvantaged those of low socioeconomic status, recording, for example, that when social marketing campaigns dominated, only 2.9% of those children in the "most poor" category used ITNs. By contrast, 66.3% of children in the same category used the intervention in 2006–2007, following free mass distribution campaigns.[91] The "most poor" group also had higher coverage levels under free distribution compared to the "least poor." "In recent years, there has been a consensus among national ministries of health, development partners, and other stakeholders that access to health interventions should be made pro-poor," Noor and his colleagues wrote. "To the best of our knowledge this is the first time in Africa that a large-scale public health intervention, covering millions of people, has preferentially reached the most-poor quintiles of a community when compared to the least poor."[92]

The team also tracked child mortality among the cohort to link health outcomes to intervention access. Looking at their data, researchers associated ITN use among children under five with a 44% reduction in mortality over the entire study period.[93] Mortality rates declined much more in high-transmission areas of Bondo than in low-transmission areas of Makueni.[94] Of course, multiple variables, including ecological conditions and the government's adoption of new antimalarial drugs in clinics in 2006, confounded any straightforward attribution of mortality reductions to high ITN coverage. However, researchers felt that these variables had little impact on their findings and were "nevertheless confident that a substantial effect on child survival was achieved during the expansion phase" of the study. "Donor agencies should regard this as money well spent," they concluded, "and recognise that the challenge is now to maintain and increase funding to expand coverage further."[95]

The general conclusion that more people used ITNs if they could access the intervention was not shocking or novel, even if "Silicon Valley types" thought otherwise. However, malaria control programmers and researchers had only produced anecdotal evidence or evidence from small-scale projects that free bed net distribution was an effective public health strategy. This helps explain why the WHO singled out the KEMRI-Wellcome Trust study in 2007 to justify its new official position that long-lasting insecticidal nets should be distributed free or highly subsidized to all people living in areas at risk for malaria. The WHO's new director-general, Margaret Chan, touted Kenya's experience, saying, "The collaboration between the Government of Kenya, WHO, and donors serves as a model that should be replicated throughout malarious countries in Africa."[96]

It is difficult to know with certainty why the WHO mobilized the team's results to endorse free net distribution at this moment, though the organization's initial press release provides some hints. For one thing, the press release suggested that the WHO was already primed for recommending free distribution since the organization had helped Kenyan officials get funding to implement the strategy. The WHO's support also reflected its recent efforts to promote universal health coverage and universal access to maternal and child health services in response to the world's slow progress toward global health and development goals.[97] In addition, the Kenyan study also provided concrete, measurable evidence linking free distribution, increased coverage and use, and reductions in child mortality. "In Kenya, from 2004 to 2006," the release stated, "a near ten-fold increase in the number of young children sleeping under insecticide-treated mosquito nets was observed in targeted districts, resulting in 44% fewer deaths than among children not protected by nets."[98] This appeared to be "the first demonstration of the impact of large-scale distribution of insecticide treated mosquito nets under programme conditions, rather than in research settings."[99] Making explicit connections between distribution strategies and mortality rates could help secure investments from donors concerned with accounting for the health impact of their dollars. "This data from Kenya ends the debate about how to deliver long-lasting insecticidal nets," Arata Kochi, head of the WHO's Global Malaria Control Programme, proclaimed. "No longer should the safety and well-being of your family be based upon whether you are rich or poor."[100] ITNs, rather, should be universally available tools and in particular, health tools for Africa's poor populations.

Domesticating ITNs in the Age of Free Distribution

Following the WHO's recommendation that countries strive for universal coverage with insecticide-treated nets (specifically long-lasting nets) through free mass distribution campaigns, major donor agencies embraced this approach. The Global Fund, which had awarded Kenya the funds to test free net distribution back in 2004, gave the Ministry of Health grant money to initiate a national distribution campaign in 2008–2009. The United States and its new President's Malaria Initiative (PMI) contributed to the endeavor as well in 2007, giving an additional $6.1 million. Drawing on funds from these and other partners, the Ministry of Health began to run free mass campaigns every three years—the low-range estimate for the life span of a long-lasting insecticidal net. PSI remained active in the country's ITN programming, continuing to promote use of the intervention through social marketing messaging and helping coordinate routine net distribution for pregnant women and infants in between mass campaigns. By the mid-2010s, household ownership of ITNs hovered between 60% and 70% nationally. However, this proportion has been dropping since 2017, and the disruptions caused by the COVID-19 pandemic hastened the decline.[101]

Undoubtedly, free mass distribution campaigns have accelerated the domestication of ITNs in Kenya, especially among populations living on the eastern coast and around Lake Victoria who are often targeted in these activities. On the whole, malaria cases and mortality rates have declined as well, partly due to the widespread use of ITNs, though it is difficult to make direct or exact attributions. Rural communities have also incorporated ITN campaigns into local social infrastructures. Community health workers and other local authorities walk around to homesteads as part of these campaigns to count how many nets each house should receive, the ideal being one net for every two people. They also tell people where to pick up the nets—usually a health facility, school, or local administrator's office. This system has facilitated net distribution in rural, outlying areas where populations are spread out and do not visit health clinics frequently. "The system they [the government] have started using of distributing the nets . . . has brought us far," one woman in Nyamache told me. "Now whether rich or poor, all have got the nets."[102]

Despite noticeable reductions in malaria since the mid-2000s, free mass campaigns have not solved all problems with Kenya's ITN activities. Distribution within campaigns is still uneven. I conducted my fieldwork in Nyamache during a free mass campaign. A few people complained that they did not receive enough nets during this distribution—some expecting one net for each person, some claiming to have received less than one net for every two people. One elderly widow had not even heard nets were being distributed, having stayed in her home, sick, for weeks. Residents of other areas shared similar complaints. "There is a lot of mischief, or let me call it a gap, in the distribution of the nets," a woman from Nyawita explained. "You realize that whenever they record your names that you have six members in your households, but later on you're only given two nets. Sometimes you'll find that your name was not even on that list." Asked if she knew why these hitches existed, the woman responded, "It is hard to tell where that mistake is coming from because the people who record the names, the community health worker, when you ask them they say, 'I recorded your name.' The hospital says 'your name is not on the list.'"[103] Mass campaigns patched many holes in bed net distribution, but certainly not all.

Free mass distribution campaigns geared toward universal coverage have also accelerated the spread of pyrethroid resistance among common *Anopheles* mosquito species—a development that experts have anticipated for decades.[104] Manufacturers have been innovating with the technology to slow insecticide resistance, including dual active ingredient nets that pair pyrethroids with other insecticides and nets that incorporate piperonyl butoxide as a synergist to block or delay mosquitoes' metabolism of the pyrethroid insecticide.[105] The PMI and other agencies have begun to procure these new generation nets for Kenya and other African countries, though these are more expensive than previous models. Since most African manufacturers do not have the capabilities for making high-quality long-lasting nets, much less new generation synergist nets, at scale, they will need to continue relying heavily on imported products and thus, on functioning global supply chains.[106] Even with sophisticated technical improvements, however, some users find that their bed nets do not always last for the three-year period between distribution campaigns, particularly in rural areas where nibbling rats, cooking fires, and normal wear and tear routinely threaten the physical integrity of the fabric.

Unsurprisingly, many people continue to use ITNs to fence their gardens, dry maize, catch fish, and perform other tasks of daily living. They use the tool to help earn an income, feed their families, and maintain healthy homes, though not in ways that policy makers and malaria control advocates had initially imagined. It is unclear to what extent free mass campaigns have contributed to these patterns of use, especially since data from other parts of the continent suggest that those who acquire nets outside free campaigns also use old, worn nets for purposes other than blocking mosquitoes.[107] Nonetheless, Ministry of Health officials and NGO partners do try to police such alternative uses to maintain malaria control practices as well as to avoid negative publicity around the provision of free nets. This surveillance is not foolproof, as one community health worker told me, because people often just temporarily remove bed net-garden fences when they know authorities are coming around. Persistent conditions of economic precarity, including threats of drought, food insecurity, and disease remain in many of Kenya's malaria-endemic regions. Residents have repurposed this simple, flexible malaria control device to mitigate against these threats.

The proliferation of nonbiodegradable ITN products and packaging has also had a noticeable impact on the environment. Some fish populations in Lake Victoria, for instance, have been reduced because they are caught in small-holed bed nets before reaching maturity and reproducing.[108] Pyrethroids embedded in long-lasting nets are also toxic to fish and aquatic life in high doses. This has added to concerns of food insecurity in lakeside communities. Since ITNs remain one of the few financially accessible, effective, and donor-supported malaria control interventions on the market, however, they will continue to become further integrated into the Kenyan landscape—both inside and outside people's homes.

While conducting fieldwork in western Kenya I met people who had a variety of ideas about and experiences with using ITNs. My research assistant, Molly, told me about how she and her siblings used to play and pretend their bed nets were small houses or forts. She admitted that, initially, she had no idea why anyone would investigate the history of an object that seemed to be, and had always been, such a commonplace piece of household furniture. On the other hand, the late Kenyan entomologist and former director of KEM-RI's Centre for Global Health Research, John Vulule, told me he did not sleep under a bed net at all. Yes, he was an adult who lived in a malaria-endemic area of Kenya for decades, and a bout of malaria for him would not be as serious as for someone with little or compromised immunity. Still, it seemed surprising to me that a malaria expert who researched this intervention for many years would not use the widely touted tool. Severe or fatal malaria, Vulule explained, is a product of poverty. If he or his family members came down with malaria, he could easily afford and access medicines. He could afford to buy additional bed nets for his children if they needed them. Those less fortunate do not have money for medical services or commodities; they can often only afford to build houses ventilated with permanent, wide-open eaves that invite in malaria-carrying mosquitoes. Due in part to Kenya-based activities and research from the 2000s, a significant proportion of Kenya's poorest citizens do have access to ITNs. More than pulling people out of poverty, though, this former luxury item has become domesticated as a health technology of poor populations.

Conclusion

Lessons for Global Health and Malaria Control in a Precarious Age

More than two decades have passed since the first summit to Roll Back Malaria in Africa. Over this period, governments, nongovernmental agencies, and private organizations have helped distribute more than 2 billion insecticide-treated nets (primarily long-lasting insecticidal nets) across Africa and the global south. This includes over 200 million nets delivered in 2020 alone, despite disruptions wrought by the COVID-19 pandemic.[1] Since 2000, the proportion of households in sub-Saharan Africa that own ITNs has increased substantially, from around 5% in 2000 to an estimated 65% in 2020. Not everyone who owns a net also sleeps under it regularly. Levels of ITN use have nonetheless also risen to over 40% of the region's population.[2] To be sure, African malaria control programs have not relied solely on ITNs to reduce malaria rates over the past two decades, but this intervention has been the most widespread and accessible among at-risk populations. Despite the spread of pyrethroid resistance, ITNs remain the largest single item in most African malaria control budgets and are commonly listed first among preventive interventions in malaria reports.

This book has examined how and why ITNs became a cornerstone of global malaria control in the twenty-first century and what the consequences of that development were. What was originally a cheap stopgap measure for twin public health and economic crises, and an imagined tool for building up "community-based" primary health care services in Africa during the 1980s, eventually transformed into the lead prong of a donor-driven effort to rid the world of malaria. At some points, in fact, it seemed that at-risk populations were receiving "nothing but nets." The parallel increase in ITN distribution and general decline of malaria rates on the continent (with some exceptions) may lead one to believe that the medical efficacy of this technology alone clinched its place in our current malaria control arsenal. Indeed, some researchers have attributed 68% of averted clinical malaria cases in Africa from 2000 to 2015 to ITNs.[3]

But the story of ITNs' ascendance is not that simple. A myriad of political, economic, and social factors shaped this object's journey as much as the development of pyrethroid insecticides or scientific demonstrations of efficacy. The political desirability and economic exigencies of decentralized, low-cost health care solutions in poor, rural areas prompted and informed initial scientific trials of bed nets in Africa. The social worlds and ecologies of African research sites, meanwhile, influenced how scientists produced scientific knowledge about ITNs and what knowledge they produced. Bed net users across the continent also had a profound effect on the development of ITN technology, such as the move to embed insecticide into net fibers during the manufacturing process in response to low net treatment rates. One cannot, in other words, wholly separate the science and technology from the context in which they were produced. Nor did scientific consensus alone dictate when and why this health intervention was deployed. Some academics and health officials actually encouraged African populations to adopt ITNs before scientists demonstrated that the tool could save lives in areas of moderate or intense malaria transmission. Others, particularly major donor agencies, were slow to promote or financially support the intervention immediately following the publication of scientific results. The practice of evidence-based global health is not necessarily this neat linear process in which research begets policy, which then translates into public health action.

Similarly, while technical constraints in malaria control—including the backlash against insecticide-spraying campaigns, rise of chloroquine resistance, and stalled efforts to produce an effective vaccine—certainly shaped the trajectory of ITNs, so too did broader developments in the field of global health. The growing privatization, decentralization, and corporatization of global health, and donors' heavy reliance on randomized controlled trials and cost-effectiveness calculations to rationalize health investments since 1980 were especially influential. Major donor agencies, for example, cited the suitability of ITNs for private sector distribution channels in their decision to support intervention and malaria control more generally, alongside statistical results from efficacy trials. This confluence of political, economic, and epistemic change that coalesced at the turn of the twenty-first century significantly influenced the rise of ITNs. At the same time, the transformation of nets into a poster child for evidence-based global health contributed to the entrenchment of these changes in our contemporary global health enterprise. Large-scale, community randomized controlled trials of nonpharmaceutical interventions have proliferated since the 1990s; ITN trials not only demonstrated the viability of this experimental framework in resource-constrained environments but also laid the groundwork for similar research. This book, then, is not simply a history of malaria control in the late twentieth and twenty-first centuries; it is also a look at how infrastructures of evidence-based global health have taken shape, as told through the biography of a quintessential evidence-based technology.

Even though African populations have played a significant role in the development of ITNs and global malaria control, they have not had an equal say in global health decision making. Beginning in the early 1990s, for instance, African researchers and health officials proposed bed net innovations and alternatives to better tailor the intervention to specific local or national contexts. They stressed a desire for malaria control strategies that African populations and health systems could eventually sustain on their own, albeit with initial help from donors given their countries' immense economic constraints under structural adjustment. As development agencies, nongovernmental organizations, and philanthropists became increasingly involved in malaria control activities during the twenty-first century, ideas changed regarding how African countries could achieve self-sufficiency and whether that was a main priority. Hopes of integrating ITNs into national and village-level infrastructures, and building up bed net manufacturing on the continent, gave way to plans to market nets and insecticide on a large scale. While marketing efforts aimed to transfer the burden of ITN delivery to the private sector, and thus relieve governments and donors of this task, this narrowly economic vision of sustainability failed to significantly affect intervention coverage levels or malaria rates. As a result, donors operating through the logic of humanitarian biomedicine began to prioritize the mass transfer of imported ITN commodities.[4] Early hopes of building up bed net manufacturing on the continent remain unrealized. At-risk populations informed the evolution of ITN distribution strategies but have had little say in whether nets are their preferred malaria control method. Such power dynamics are not unique to the case of ITNs or to the African continent but are characteristic of the field of global health more generally.[5]

This biography of ITNs highlights some pitfalls of neglecting the perspectives of those affected by the health issue in question. Many obstacles faced by programmers in getting ITNs to work as intended during the twenty-first century were not new. People involved in early bed net trials had experienced many of these challenges years before Roll Back Malaria leaders decided to scale up the intervention. Surveys of African research participants during the 1980s and 1990s revealed that those most at risk for malaria either could not afford bed nets or considered bed nets less important than other household expenditures such as food or school fees. These surveys also revealed that the links between ITN use and protection from malaria were not always obvious to intended users, who were asked to sleep under a pungent-smelling, often uncomfortable sheet of fabric previously seen as a luxury item. ITNs, researchers stressed, were not suitable for everyone everywhere, including places where mosquitoes did not feed indoors or where bed nets did not fit in people's houses or sleeping spaces.

It is no surprise, then, that selling ITNs through cookie-cutter social marketing campaigns did not increase coverage substantially among intended users during the early years of Roll Back Malaria. Underappreciated gender dimensions of household relations, malaria risk, and poverty complicated these campaigns, which aimed to reach mothers as caregivers and beneficiaries in their own right. African health officials and bed net manufacturers also recognized the precariousness of relying on external donors for malaria control interventions, yet the particular capitalist structures of global health and development (global commodity funds, pay-for-performance funding models, public-private partnerships favoring private agencies from wealthy countries) encouraged this dependence. Africans' experiences with ITNs illuminate some of the shortcomings of using individualized commodity solutions to tackle malaria on the continent, especially the inability of such interventions to address underlying economic inequalities that make it difficult for people to avoid infection, access necessary health care, or maintain malaria control strategies long term. Understanding their experiences, needs, and constraints, and how these have been shaped by the structures of our contemporary global health enterprise can contribute immensely to understanding persistent global health challenges.

Although it is difficult to measure the public health impact of ITNs with any accuracy, it is clear that they have made a substantial difference in the fight against malaria. Before the disruptions wrought by the COVID-19 pandemic, malaria deaths in Africa had decreased by over a third, from an estimated 840,000 in 2000 to 534,000 in 2019.[6] Considering that at-risk populations have not had steady access to effective and affordable antimalarial drugs over this period, particularly before the widespread adoption of artemisinin combination therapy as a first-line treatment option in the mid-2000s, it is difficult to dispute that ITNs played an important role in this decline. This is to say nothing of the critical part that the intervention played in efforts to draw international attention and funding to malaria control in Africa at the end of the 1990s, mobilizing various groups around the goal of rolling back malaria on the continent.

Developments over the past five to ten years, however, have threatened the viability of using ITNs for malaria control in the long term. As malaria experts predicted as far back as the early 1990s, many species of *Anopheles* mosquito have started to become resistant to pyrethroid insecticides used in ITNs. The mass, universal distribution of the technology after 2008 greatly accelerated rates of insecticide resistance. Researchers and manufacturers are trying to innovate with the technology to slow resistance and maintain the tool's effectiveness. Companies have begun to manufacture long-lasting nets that incorporate piperonyl butoxide (PBO) as a synergist to block or delay mosquitoes' metabolism of pyrethroids. Some have also started making dual active ingredient nets that pair pyrethroids with other insecticides that work via a different mode of action. About a quarter of the nets delivered to Africa in 2020 were either PBO or dual active ingredient nets, though it still is unclear how quickly these new generation products can be scaled up to replace those currently in use.[7] In addition, researchers have started testing rectangular nets with a flap on top coated in a nonpyrethroid insecticide that is supposed to repel or kill mosquitoes as they move side to side above the net. Others have even begun coating nets with antimalarial drug compounds to interrupt the development of parasites in mosquitoes' guts.[8] However, many of these and similar innovations are still in the testing phase.[9] And while scientists have finally produced a long-awaited malaria vaccine (RTS,S/AS01)—for which bed nets originally functioned as a placeholder of sorts— it is only moderately efficacious even after the four required doses.

Major donors to malaria control in Africa have also started reducing their contributions. In light of this retraction, and realizing the threat this poses to health gains, the World Health Organization (WHO) has pushed African governments to take on more of the financial responsibility for malaria control in their countries. Since many governments still cannot afford to subsidize the recommended arsenal of malaria control tools—including nets, drugs, selective indoor residual spraying, and now the vaccine—they and their expatriate partners have begun to invest more in private sector delivery of ITNs. Since ITN manufacturing did not develop substantially on the continent, governments must still import these products. New generation nets that address the growing problem of insecticide resistance, such as synergist nets, will be more expensive than those currently in use. This will place an extra burden on those countries where insecticide-resistance is already high. Some of the countries suffering with the highest malaria burdens are also some of the poorest, making the shift to country-led malaria control difficult. Even before the outbreak of the COVID-19 pandemic, gains in malaria control had begun to plateau, with some countries in the region actually experiencing increases in malaria case and mortality rates.[10]

The outbreak of the COVID-19 pandemic added an extra obstacle not just to reducing malaria in Africa, but to simply maintaining current malaria rates. Many countries instituted lockdown measures to help contain the pandemic, which interfered with ITN distribution during 2020. The pandemic also disrupted the global supply chain of health commodities as well as health service delivery in malaria-endemic countries, including case management with antimalarial drugs. Malaria mortality in sub-Saharan Africa increased from an estimated 534,000 to 602,000 from 2019 to 2020. The full consequences of this pandemic remain to be seen, not only on people's health and access to health care but also on countries' ability and willingness to fund malaria control efforts at the level necessary to maintain health gains. The escalating climate crisis, which has led to severe droughts, flooding, and crop failures across the continent in recent years, will exacerbate food insecurity, poverty, and malaria transmission. The consequences of this for malaria control efforts remain to be seen as well. Although aspects of these current complications are unique, none of them are entirely new. Some of these same issues, in fact, arose following the end of the WHO's Malaria Eradication Programme—including increasing insecticide resistance, the detrimental health effects of declining funding for malaria programs, and the disruption of a novel pandemic (HIV/AIDS). Then, as now, malaria rates around the world dropped significantly only to bounce back in certain areas, particularly in places where reductions in malaria were not necessarily accompanied by gains in social and economic development among the most vulnerable populations. And while health and development leaders have linked malaria control to poverty reduction in the twenty-first century, much as health officials linked malaria eradication to economic development in the 1950s and 1960s, ITNs have not proved sufficient for pulling people out of poverty. Many are still vulnerable to increasing disease rates in unstable economic and environmental conditions. The infrastructure and machinery of global health has largely left this vulnerability intact.

No small part of this is due to the fact that global health programs today run largely on the distribution of health commodities, such as drugs, vaccines, diagnostic tests, and personal preventive measures like ITNs. Still, a majority of these commodities are manufactured by multinational companies in wealthy countries, or at least those that do not constitute the primary market for these products. Low-income countries struggling with disease burdens must pay to import these goods or, as is common, rely on external donors to help procure them. The COVID-19 pandemic throws the pitfalls of this system into sharp relief with the disruption of commodity supply chains and distribution. Even before the pandemic, however, stagnating (and even reversing) rates of malaria in high-burden countries illustrated the limitations of relying on commodities to solve this complex, long-standing public health problem.

The fact that individualized commodities, particularly pharmaceuticals, have become such a substantial part of global health programming is not a novel insight. Few, however, have explored how these interventions fit into a broader economy of global health goods, an economy in which cost-per-life-saved has become enshrined as a key metric and source of value.[11] Claims that ITNs saved lives for relatively little money, alongside the intervention's suitability for decentralized and private sector distribution, proved critical to patrons' financial and political support. Randomized controlled trial and cost-effectiveness data showed nets to be comparable, even competitive, with other tools of child survival. Since child survival was an important metric of economic development in the late twentieth and twenty-first centuries, ITNs seemed quite valuable. Groups—ranging from wealthy development agencies and global health philanthropies to individual donors to bed net charities—

paid to send nets to save lives on the basis of this value. While ITNs did not begin as "global health commodities," this identity was crucial to their widespread uptake as a primary malaria control intervention.

ITNs did not just spur new groups and people to get involved in global health programming; the already-shifting makeup of global health participants also contributed to the intervention's wide proliferation. Amid a severe economic crisis, development banks, economists, private and nongovernmental agencies, and philanthrocapitalists came to play a larger role in global health decision making, while the influence of internationally representative bodies, such as the WHO and UN, declined.[12] At the same time, wealthy countries increasingly looked to the private and nongovernmental sectors to supply and distribute global health interventions in low-income settings. Those with the ability to finance global health activities in the late twentieth century prioritized economic efficiency and accountability in their investments, seeking to make the biggest health impact with the least money. They also stressed the benefits of market-based governance, often prioritizing expertise in marketing, corporate management, and microeconomics over skill in public health or health systems. Using biostatistics and econometrics as markers of public health effectiveness—which provide some, but not necessarily all of the picture—they have procured and circulated health commodities in bulk under the banner of saving lives and alleviating poverty. As the history of ITNs illustrates, this approach is not a sustainable form of global health intervention and, at times, it ignores important insights of locally situated public health experts and affected populations.

It appears that ITNs will continue to play a major role in malaria control, despite the spread of insecticide resistance and the recent development of a malaria vaccine. But as the world moves forward with new medical and public health innovations, it is important not to lose sight of these objects' history. The ways in which health technologies take shape—both materially and conceptually—and the ways they evolve alongside health systems affects how people later apply them in practice. Ignoring the initial challenges of getting health technologies to function as intended, or the conditions shown to be necessary to their effective use, can hinder successful intervention. Likewise, ignoring the perspectives of those most familiar with the technology and the context in which it will be applied can inhibit public health efforts.

After all, new health interventions are not introduced in isolation; they must be integrated into extant political, economic, sociocultural, epidemiological, and technological landscapes at the same time that they reshape those terrains. Therefore, attending to the history of "evidence-based" technologies in global health is not merely an academic exercise; it is a method that might be useful in crafting more effective global health programs.

Acknowledgments

Although I appear as the sole author of this book, so many people shaped my thinking, research, and writing as I completed it. To them, I am deeply indebted. Any errors or omissions in the book are my responsibility alone.

I will never be able to express my full appreciation for the ongoing guidance and support of Randall Packard. He has been there for me through this entire process, reading draft after draft of chapters as well as the full manuscript as this project took shape. I benefited immensely from his wisdom, mentorship, and editorial eye. I could not have written this book without him.

I also could not have completed this book without the help of my research assistant, Molly Omany, who was an important guide and friend for me while I conducted fieldwork in Kenya in 2015 and 2016. I will never be able to document just how much I learned from her. Simon Kariuki was instrumental in providing me with institutional support at the Kenya Medical Research Institute-Centre for Global Health Research in Kisumu. I thank the National Commission for Science, Technology and Innovation and Maseno University for additional institutional support that allowed me to do this work. Sam Onyango, Lillian and the team at Halo-Kenya in Asembo, and the community health workers in Asembo, Gem, Bondo, and Gucha facilitated my research in essential ways. Bernard Okal, Judy Kiprop, and the Bakari family were important teachers for me, not just in Dholuo and KiSwahili but in the history and culture of Kenya as well. I appreciate the wonderful reception I received working in Kenya and feel incredibly fortunate to have met so many amazing people while there.

I also want to thank the many people who agreed to be interviewed and share their time and insights for this study. The details and perspectives they provided helped me understand the history of global health at a level I would not have been able to access otherwise. I especially want to acknowledge Don de Savigny, Simon Kariuki, S. Patrick Kachur, Steve Lindsay, Jo Lines, Penelope Phillips-Howard, and Bob Snow, who were excellent hosts and provided important contacts and materials for the project. Numerous archivists and librarians helped me during the research process, including Reynald Erard at the WHO Archives, Amanda Leinberger at the UN Archives, Shiri Alon and staff at the World Bank Archives, and Claire Frankland at the Archives of the London School of Hygiene and Tropical Medicine. Their efforts were essential to my completion of this project.

I could not have asked for a better intellectual home than the Johns Hopkins History of Medicine Department, where I did the bulk of this research. I benefitted immensely from my interactions with members of the department over the many years I spent there. Yulia Frumer, Jeremy Greene, Clara Han, and Graham Mooney helped me think more broadly about global health, particularly about technology, materiality, and space. The other members of the Critical Global Health Seminar also provided me with a valuable forum for discussing and thinking about the nature of this enterprise. Sara Berry, Jessica Levy, Dan Todes, and Alice Wiemers were key to the development of my thinking on the history of capitalism and development. Members of the African Seminar provided many useful suggestions about how to integrate African history and the history of global health. The late Pier Larson helped me tremendously in thinking about this project as an African history and was a very careful and supportive reader of my work. I regret that he will not be able to see this in its final form.

I had the good fortune to spend a year at the Beckman Center of the Chemical Heritage Foundation (now Science History Institute) in 2016–2017 to work on this research. Carin Berkowitz contributed some very useful feedback on my work and the publishing process more generally. I truly appreciate her guidance. My colleagues at the Beckman Center and in the Philadelphia history of science community, including Thomas Apel, Nicholas Bonneau, Cari Casteel, Nicole Cook, Joe Martin, Elisabeth Moreau, Agnieszka Rec, Jean-Olivier Richard, and Frank Zelko, offered additional help during the writing and editing process. I thank the Beckman Center and the Science History Institute for generous support.

I was also incredibly lucky to have had the support of Cedars-Sinai Medical Center and my colleagues in the Program in the History of Medicine there during this process. Leon Fine has provided me with a wonderful institutional home. He also offered useful advice and perspectives from the world of biomedical sciences that helped me in completing the book. Both he and Gideon Manning have always been encouraging of my work and process, and

I am grateful for their continued guidance. I also benefited from many conversations with colleagues in the Cedars-Sinai Program in the History of Medicine, including Devon Golaszewski, Peiting Li, Melissa Lo, Rena Selya, and Sari Siegel, as well as attendees at the Biomedical and Translational Science Seminar Series. Their questions were incredibly useful as I honed my writing and argument.

Coming to Cedars-Sinai also put me in touch with many other scholars in and around Los Angeles whose comments, suggestions, and encouragement shaped this project. My discussions with Soraya de Chadarevian, Ted Porter, and Mary Terrall at UCLA greatly informed my thinking about global health science and offered valuable guidance. I appreciated many conversations with other colleagues at UCLA working on the history of science and medicine, including Amir Alexander, Scottie Buehler, Iris Clever, Bob Frank, Jacob Green, Chien Ling Liu Zeleny, Josh McGuffie, Marcia Meldrum, Bharat Venkat, and Norton Wise. I thank them for helping me feel welcome in Los Angeles. I learned a lot about the history of global health from Ippolytos Kalofonos and from lecturing in his Introduction to Global Health course. The students in my own courses on the History of Global Health Technology and the History of Colonial and Postcolonial Science and Technology pushed me to think about my topic in new ways. I am particularly grateful to Tiffany Han and Sahej Verma for thinking through the globalization of biomedicine with me. I would also like to thank Cathy Gere and Dana Simmons for their encouragement and guidance.

So many scholars proved invaluable to me as I wrote this book, not only as readers and editors but also as friends and mentors. I benefited immensely from my friendship and conversations with Penelope Hardy, Lisa Haushofer, Seth LeJacq, Misha Mintz-Roth, and Felix Reitmann. They were especially helpful as I navigated the process of writing a first book. Ken Alder, Abena Osseo-Asare, Thomas Cousins, David Jones, Andrew Lakoff, Marissa Mika, and Dora Vargha helped me think about the role of technologies in global health. I am incredibly grateful to Mari Webel and Anne Pollock, who read and commented on chapters from the book. They saw opportunities for insights in an Africa-centered narrative of global health that I may not have picked up on otherwise. Mari also organized a working group around the topic of neglected tropical diseases, which has been the perfect network for me and my intellectual interests. I appreciate the insights I have gleaned from João Nunes, Noémi Tousignant, Samantha Vanderslott, and Viona Sari as part of that group. Claire Gherini has been a truly amazing editor and friend, especially in the final stages of the writing process. I absolutely could not have completed this book without the suggestions and support of Julia Cummiskey and Heidi Morefield, who not only read some of my chapters but provided motivation and inspiration at key moments.

I benefited from comments on my work in numerous venues, including audiences at the meetings of the African Studies Association, American Association for the History of Medicine, History of Science Society, Sam Houston State Medical Humanities lecture series, Society for the History of Technology, UCLA History of Science Colloquium, and Society for the Social Studies of Science (4S). The STS in Africa working group at 4S in Sydney was a great venue for developing my ideas about science and technology on the continent. I am also grateful to all those who provided comments on a draft article from this project through the Consortium for the History of Science, Technology, and Medicine working group on Medicine and Health. Portions of this research appeared in that article, "Marketing Malaria Control: Nets, Neoliberalism and a New Approach to Fighting Malaria," *Social History of Medicine* (published online, 2022). I thank Oxford University Press for permission to reprint that material. I also thank my editor, Matt McAdam, anonymous readers, and the entire team at Johns Hopkins University Press for helping to improve this book and bring it to fruition.

Finally, I would like to thank my family for their unconditional love and support. My parents, Janet and Ron, have always been there for me. They continue to be among my most important teachers and supporters. And I could not have done any of this without my husband, Austin, who has given so much of his time and energy to make this project happen. He has trudged through my writing at numerous stages, reading this book in its entirety at least once and portions of it many times over. He has been my rock throughout this process, including through the COVID-19 pandemic and the birth of our first child, Damian. He has always been my biggest fan and has helped me keep going through the most difficult times. There are no words to express how lucky I feel to have him by my side as my life partner.

Notes

Introduction. Making Evidence-Based Global Health in Africa

1. United Nations Foundation, "NothingButNets.net."

2. United to Beat Malaria, "Our Impact."

3. Reilly, "Nothing But Nets."

4. For more on evidence-based practices in global health, see Adams, "Evidence-based global public health."

5. Packard, *Making of a Tropical Disease*; Cueto, "Return to the magic bullet?"; and Webb, *Long Struggle against Malaria*.

6. For an in-depth analysis of this argument, see Redfield, "Bioexpectations."

7. Notable exceptions include Redfield, "Vital mobility"; and Greene, "Making medicines essential." For analyses covering the period before the 1980s, see Bhattacharya, *Expunging Variola*; and Vargha, *Polio across the Iron Curtain*.

8. For other examples of how African settings and scientists informed seemingly universal scientific knowledge, see Schumaker, *Africanizing Anthropology*; Heaton, *Black Skin, White Coats*; and Pollock, *Synthesizing Hope*.

9. Kopytoff, "Cultural biography of things"; Daston, *Biographies of Scientific Objects*; Whyte, Van der Geest, and Hardon, *Social Lives of Medicines*; and Takeshita, *Global Biopolitics of the IUD*.

10. Or, as Uli Beisel has termed them, "humanitarian goods." Beisel, "Markets and mutations."

11. For an overview of this history, see Packard, *History of Global Health*.

12. Brown, Cueto, and Fee, "World Health Organization."

13. Adams, "Evidence-based global public health."

14. Kramer, "Embedding capitalism," 341.

15. Baird, "Malaria control by commodities," 593.

16. I invoke the idea of desirable utility here to suggest that a commodity or object does not always have a fixed utility for everyone. Different people may use the same object to satisfy different needs. For more on this approach to Karl Marx's concept of use value, see Burke, *Lifebuoy Men, Lux Women*, 8.

17. King, "Security, disease, commerce."

18. Beisel, "Markets and mutations."

19. Some of these issues are also explored in Baird, "Malaria control by commodities."

20. Kopytoff describes objects as having many biographies—for example, physical, economic, and social—in which that object can take on different meanings. I draw on this insight to look at different domains (or in Kopytoff's words, biographies) of the life of ITNs but in areas more specific to public health objects and less applicable to objects in general. Kopytoff, "Cultural biography of things," 68. For an example of a biography exploring the many facets or identities of a person, see Golinski, *Experimental Self*.

21. Although I use "insecticide-treated nets" and "ITNs" throughout the book, the technology itself has not remained the same over the period covered in this history, including in terms of fabric, shape, size, and insecticide type. Most notably, before the twenty-first century the nets and insecticide were separate items, and one had to coat nets with insecticide every six months to maintain them as insecticide-treated nets. During the twenty-first century, manufacturers began embedding net fibers with insecticide, so people increasingly received them ready-made as long-lasting insecticide-treated nets. When it is important to the discussion, I make distinctions between ordinary (untreated) bed nets, insecticide-treated bed nets (ITNs), insecticide-treated curtains, and long-lasting insecticidal nets. Otherwise, I use "insecticide-treated net," "ITN," or "bed net" as a general term for the intervention.

22. Daston, *Biography of Scientific Objects*.

Chapter 1. The Scientific Object

1. Daston, *Biographies of Scientific Objects*.

2. Clark and Fujimura, "What tools?" 5.

3. Adams, "Evidence-based global public health."

4. Graboyes, "'Malaria imbroglio.'"

5. Molyneux and Gramiccia, *Garki Project*.

6. Carpenter et al., *Malaria*, 44.

7. Webb, *Long Struggle against Malaria*, 107.

8. Webb, *Long Struggle against Malaria*, 101–3.

9. Walsh and Warren, "Selective primary health care."

10. For more on the history of the concept and promotion of "appropriate technology" in international development, see Morefield, "'More with less.'"

11. Harrison Spencer, "The Global Strategy for Malaria Control within Primary Health Care as Recommended by the 18th Committee on Malaria," July 1986, WHO Archives, Geneva, File M2-370-21, Jacket 5.

12. Dr. H. Cárdenas Gutiérrez, "Organizational aspects of the epidemiological approach to malaria control," paper presented at the 19th Expert Committee on Malaria in Geneva, November 6–15, 1989, WHO Archives, File M2-81-19, Jacket 1.

13. Webb, *Long Struggle against Malaria*, 114.

14. P. G. Janssens, "Comments on 'Guidelines on malaria control in different geographical areas,'" 1983, 7, WHO Archives, File M2-374-13, Jacket 3.

15. Packard, *Making of a Tropical Disease*, 164.

16. Beausoleil, "Review of present antimalaria activities."

17. Packard, *Making of a Tropical Disease*, 174.

18. Lindsay and Gibson, "Bednets revisited."

19. Winslow, *On the Preservation of Health*, 42.

20. Harper et al., "Malaria and other insect-borne diseases"; Blagoveschensky et al., "Investigation of new repellants"; and Wenren and Henglin, *Zhongguo nüeji de fangzhi yu yanjiu*. I thank Yubin Shen for pointing me to the Wenren and Henglin source and providing information on net use in China. I also thank James Flowers for helping me with translation.

21. Davis, *Banned*, 195–200.

22. Lin, "Bednets treated with pyrethroids," 67.

23. Self, "Perspective piece."

24. WHO Expert Committee on Vector Biology and Control, "Integrated vector control."

25. Zu-Jie, "Malaria situation in the People's Republic of China."

26. Zuzi et al., "Mosquito nets."

27. Zuzi et al., "Mosquito nets." In some places, such as Sichuan Province, they sprayed nets with insecticide.

28. Lengeler, Cattani, and de Savigny, *Net Gain*, 59, 91.

29. WHO Expert Committee on Vector Biology and Control, "Integrated vector control."

30. For more on the dominance of entomologists in international malaria control after World War II, see Packard, *Making of a Tropical Disease*.

31. Port and Boreham, "Effect of bed nets."

32. Derriet et al., "Evaluation," 10.

33. Lines et al., "Tests of repellent," 9.

34. WHO Expert Committee on Vector Biology and Control, "Resistance of vectors."

35. WHO Scientific Group on Vector Control in Primary Health Care, "Vector Control in Primary Health Care," 12.

36. Brian Greenwood, interview with author. The MRC provided its laboratories in The Gambia with roughly $150,000 per year for bed net studies during the 1980s. Brian Greenwood, "Trial of permethrin treated bed nets in The Gambia," proposal for Special Programme for Research and Training in Tropical Diseases (TDR) Director's Initiative Fund, submitted Feb 19, 1985, WHO Archives, File T-16-181-M2-A-60.

37. Greenwood, interview with author.

38. Greenwood et al., "Mortality and morbidity."

39. Bob Snow, interview with author.

40. Bradley et al., "Bed-nets (mosquito-nets) and morbidity," 206.

41. Phillipe Ranque did a small trial to test the clinical effects of deltamethrin-treated bed nets shortly after this survey in 1983 and found lower splenomegaly in children sleeping under nets. However, the small scale of the trial made it difficult to determine whether pyrethroid-treated nets had any significant effect on malaria morbidity. Ranque et al., "Use of mosquito nets."

42. H. Carlsson in Guinea-Bissau, reported in Bradley et al., "Bed-nets (mosquito-nets) and morbidity," 204.

43. Bradley et al., "Bed-nets (mosquito-nets) and morbidity," 207.

44. Brandt and Gardner, "Antagonism and accommodation." The difference in these types of approaches to malaria are discussed in Baird, "Malaria control by commodities."

45. Greenwood, "Trial of permethrin treated bed nets."

46. Weisz and Tousignant, "International health research," 372.

47. Snow, Rowan, and Greenwood, "Trial of permethrin-treated bed nets."

48. Snow, Rowan, and Greenwood, "Trial of permethrin-treated bed nets."

49. Bermejo and Veeken, "Insecticide-impregnated bed nets."

50. For a description of this process in a different African laboratory, see Langwick, "Devils, parasites, and fierce needles."

51. MacCormack, Snow, and Greenwood, "Use of insecticide-impregnated bed nets," 211.

52. Patterson, "Net Values," 148.

53. Snow, interview with author.

54. For more on Gambian residents' suspicions of the MRC and the taking of blood, see Fairhead, Leach, and Small, "Where techno-science meets poverty."

55. Lindsay et al., "Impact of permethrin-treated bednets," 266.

56. Snow et al., "Permethrin-treated bed nets (mosquito nets)."

57. Snow et al., "Permethrin-treated bed nets (mosquito nets)," 841.

58. Brian Greenwood, Progress Report for "Effect of insecticide impregnation of bed nets on morbidity from malaria in Gambian villages, Jan 1, 1987 to June 30, 1987," 1987, WHO Archives, File T16-181-M2-A-78.

59. Letter, Dr. S. Goriup to Brian Greenwood, February 23, 1987, WHO Archives, File T16-181-M2-A-78.

60. Lindsay et al., "Impact of permethrin-treated bednets," 265.

61. Carol MacCormack, "Gambian Fula Preferences in Bed Net Use," Report for British MRC and WHO-TDR, August 1986, WHO Archives, File T16-181-M2-A-60.

62. MacCormack, "Gambian Fula Preferences."

63. Snow et al., "How best to treat bed nets," 647.

64. Snow et al., "Permethrin-treated bed nets," 841.

65. WHO Expert Committee on Vector Biology and Control, "Use of Impregnated Bednets," 6.

66. Steven Lindsay, interview with author.

67. Packard, *History of Global Health*, 256–59.

68. Alonso et al., "Accuracy of the clinical histories."

69. Greenwood et al., "Mortality and morbidity."

70. Greenwood et al., "Comparison of two drug strategies."

71. Brian M. Greenwood, Proposal to TDR for "A trial of insecticide impregnated bed nets and targetted chemoprophylaxis as a control strategy for the prevention of malaria in children within a primary health care programme," 1988, WHO Archives, File M24-181-16.

72. Letter, Dr. S Goriup to Brian Greenwood, December 7, 1987, WHO Archives, File T16-181-M2-A-78.

73. Greenwood, "Trial of insecticide impregnated bed nets."

74. Greenwood, "Trial of insecticide impregnated bed nets."

75. Brian Greenwood, Progress Report for period July 1990–June 1991 submitted to TDR, WHO Archives, File M24-181-16.

76. Lindsay, interview with author.

77. Lindsay, interview with author.

78. Histogram displayed in Alonso et al., "Effect of insecticide-treated bed nets," 1501.

79. Alonso et al., "Effect of insecticide-treated bed nets," 1501. In this case, protective efficacy refers to the percentage reduction of child mortality in the intervention group as compared to the control group after one year.

80. Brian Greenwood, Progress Report for period July 1990–June 1991.

81. Alonso et al., "Effect of insecticide-treated bed nets," 1501.

82. "Towards a Strategic Implementation Agenda on Insecticide-Impregnated Bednet Interventions," August 1994, TDR Bednet Initiative, WHO Archives, File M24-370-2.

83. Jo Lines, interview with author.

84. Lindsay, interview with author.

85. Lindsay, interview with author.

86. Bermejo and Veeken, "Insecticide-impregnated bed nets," 295.

87. Christian Lengeler, interview with author.

88. Andrew Spielman, "Research Priorities for Managing the Transmission of Vector-Borne Disease," Report for Study Group Vector Control for Malaria and Other Mosquito-Borne Diseases, WHO Archives, File Malaria1-SG- Vectors, Folder 1.

89. WHO Expert Committee on Malaria, "WHO's Malaria Control Strategy: Global Initiative, Local Action," June 24, 1992, 11, WHO Archives, File MALARIA1-SG-VECTORS-5.

90. Letter, Tore Godal to Dr. Nyi (Director of Programme Division at UNICEF), February 6, 1992, World Bank Archives, Washington, DC, File 1873045.

91. Lane, "Tore Godal."

92. Lengeler, interview with author.

93. Adams, "Metrics of the global sovereign"; and Packard, *History of Global Health*, 307–11.

94. Sommer et al., "Aceh Study Group."

95. Fred Binka, Pre-proposal submitted to TDR, "Permethrin impregnated bednets and child mortality in Ghana," September 1991, WHO Archives, File M24-181-78, Jacket 1; Dr. Lamizana and Dr. V. Pietra, Pre-proposal submitted to TDR, "Large scale trial on the efficacy of insecticide impregnated curtains in reducing malaria mortality and morbidity in children," WHO Archives, File M24-181-76, Jacket 1; and Bob Snow, Pre-proposal submitted to TDR, "Trial of the effect of impregnated bed nets on childhood mortality in Coastal Kenya," WHO Archives, File M24-181-87, Jacket 1.

96. Letter, Jackie Cattani to Dr. Lamizana and Dr. V. Pietra, November 18, 1991, WHO Archives, File M24-181-76; Letter, Jackie Cattani to Pedro Alonso, September 26, 1991, WHO Archives, File M24-181-78, Jacket 1; Lamizana and Pietra, "Large scale trial on the efficacy of insecticide impregnated curtains"; Bob Snow, Progress Report, August 7, 1994, WHO Archives, File M24-181-87, Jacket 1; and Letter, Fred Binka to Jackie Cattani, March 5, 1992, WHO Archives, File M24-181-78, Jacket 1.

97. Lamizana and Pietra, "Large scale trial on the efficacy of insecticide impregnated curtains."

98. Bob Snow, Proposal submitted to TDR, 1992, WHO Archives, File M24-181-87, Jacket 1.

99. Anne Mills, interview with author.

100. Anne Mills, Economic Evaluation of The Gambian Impregnated Bed Net Programme, 1992, WHO Archives, File M24-181-83, Jacket 1.

101. Brian Greenwood, Proposal submitted to TDR, The Gambian National Bednet Programme, 1991, WHO Archives, File M24-181-83, Jacket 1.

102. Packard, *Making of a Tropical Disease*, 166–74, 215.

103. Fred Binka, Proposal submitted to TDR, 1992, WHO Archives, File M24-181-78, Jacket 1; Lamizana and Pietra, Progress Report submitted to TDR, 1993, WHO Archives, File M24-181-76, Jacket 1; and Bob Snow, Proposal submitted to TDR, 1992, WHO Archives, File M24-181-87, Jacket 1.

104. Fred Binka, Progress Report submitted to TDR, 1992, WHO Archives, File M24-181-78, Jacket 1; and Bob Snow, Progress Report submitted to TDR, 1992, WHO Archives, File M24-181-87, Jacket 1.

105. This is similar to what Michelle Murphy has described with Knowledge, Attitudes, Practices surveys in contraceptive social marketing programs. Murphy, *Economization of Life*, 62–70.

106. Marsh et al., "Evaluating the community education programme," 281.

107. Lansina Lamizana, Progress Report submitted to TDR, 1994, WHO Archives, File M24-181-76, Jacket 1.

108. Brian Greenwood, Progress Report submitted to TDR, Gambian National Bed Net Programme, 1992, WHO Archives, File M24-181-83, Jacket 1.

109. Fred Binka, Proposal submitted to TDR, 1992, WHO Archives, File M24-181-78, Jacket 1.

110. Marsh et al., "Evaluating the community education programme," 281.

111. Bob Snow, Progress Report submitted to TDR, 1994, WHO Archives, M24-181-87, Jacket 1.

112. Bob Snow, Progress Report submitted to TDR, 1994, WHO Archives, M24-181-87, Jacket 1.

113. Brian Greenwood, Progress Report submitted to TDR, Gambian National Bednet Programme, 1993, WHO Archives, File M24-181-83, Jacket 1.

114. Habluetzel et al., "Do insecticide-treated curtains reduce all-cause child mortality?"

115. Nevill et al., "Insecticide-treated bednets."

116. Bob Snow, Progress Report submitted to TDR, 1994, WHO Archives, M24-181-87, Jacket 1.

117. Brian Greenwood, Progress Report submitted to TDR, Gambian National Bednet Programme, 1992, WHO Archives, File M24-181-83, Jacket 1.

118. Letter, Fred Binka to Jackie Cattani, February 24, 1994, WHO Archives, File M24-181-78, Jacket 2; and Bob Snow et al., "WHO funded trial of insecticide-treated bed-nets in the reduction of childhood mortality on the Kenyan Coast. Interim report on the pre-intervention year and delivery phase," August 1993, WHO Archives, File M24-181-87, Jacket 1.

119. Habluetzel et al., "Do insecticide-treated curtains reduce all-cause child mortality?"

120. Nevill et al., "Insecticide-treated bednets."

121. Nevill et al., "Insecticide-treated bednets," 144.

122. Economists calculated the cost-effectiveness of the provision of nets and insecticide at $19–85 per disability-adjusted life year averted, and $4–10 per disability-adjusted life year averted for the insecticide treatment of existing nets. These results compared favorably with many interventions, such as oral rehydration therapy and measles vaccination

(in the case of treating existing nets). Goodman, Coleman, and Mills, "Cost-effectiveness of malaria control."

123. Adams, "Evidence-based global public health."

Chapter 2. The Biomedical Technology

1. Michael Onyango, interview with author.

2. Siaya became a county under the 2010 Constitution of Kenya, which proposed a new organization of subnational units of government in the country.

3. Adams, "Metrics of the global sovereign," 34.

4. For examples of historical ethnography, see Cohen and Atieno Odhiambo, *Siaya*; Schumaker, *Africanizing Anthropology*; and Mutongi, *Worries of the Heart*.

5. *Nyamrerwa* is a Luo term initially used in Siaya to describe village health helpers who dealt with child health and midwifery and who were well known and trusted within their community. Since they could more easily communicate with pregnant women than could outside researchers, *nyamrerwa* became increasingly integrated into medical research trials dealing with maternal and child health during the 1980s. As the position of *nyamrerwa* came to encompass new duties in these trials, it became glossed as "community health worker." For more on the history of *nyamrerwa* in Siaya, see Aellah and Okoth, "'Living honourably and independently,'" 108.

6. Cohen and Odhiambo, *Siaya*, 9.

7. For recent work on this phenomenon in Africa, see Cummiskey, "Placing Global Science in Africa"; Pollock, *Synthesizing Hope*; and Webel, *Politics of Disease Control*.

8. Hutchinson, "Planning National Malaria Research"; and Elliot and Koech, *Reimagining Science*.

9. KEMRI, "Kenya Medical Research Institute," 111.

10. KEMRI, "Kenya Medical Research Institute," 112.

11. Spencer, Kaseje, and Koech, "Kenyan Saradidi Community."

12. For a more detailed discussion of KEMRI's early institutional history, including its partnership with the CDC, see Elliott and Koech, *Reimagining Science*, 94–128.

13. Sexton et al., "Permethrin-impregnated curtains," 16.

14. Beach et al., "Effectiveness of permethrin-impregnated bed nets."

15. Aggrey Oloo et al., Research proposal, "A Comparative Study of the Effect of Pyrethroid Treated Sisal Curtains and Bednets in Malaria Control," WHO Archives, Geneva, File M24-181-1, Jacket 19.

16. Dr. Jack H. P. Nyeko, Grant Proposal, "Impregnated Target Specific Nets (TAGS) in Malaria Control," WHO Archives, File M24-181-1, Jacket 25; and Mutinga et al., "Malaria prevalence and morbidity."

17. Mutinga et al., "Use of permethrin-impregnated wall cloth."

18. Weisz and Tousignant, "International health research," 370–373.

19. Bloland et al., "Longitudinal cohort study," 641.

20. Bloland et al., "Longitudinal cohort study," 641.

21. Feierman, "When physicians meet," 189.

22. USAID Bureau for Africa and Office for Sustainable Development, "USAID-DHHS Partnership in Health," 5.

23. USAID Bureau for Africa and Office for Sustainable Development, "USAID-DHHS Partnership in Health," 16.

24. William Hawley, interview with author.

25. Jack Wirima, Grant proposal, "Effect of permethrin-impregnated bed nets upon child mortality in a malaria endemic region of southern Malawi," February 1992, WHO Archives, File M24-181-1, Jacket 18.

26. Lawrence (Larry) Slutsker, interview with author.

27. Bernard Nahlen, interview with author.

28. Snow and Marsh, "Will reducing Plasmodium falciparum transmission alter malaria mortality?"

29. Packard, *Making of a Tropical Disease*, 177–216. This shift in the age profile of malaria was also seen specifically following indoor residual spraying projects in Liberia during the 1950s. Webb, "First large-scale use of synthetic insecticide," 366.

30. Feiko ter Kuile, interview with author.

31. Randall Packard, personal communication, Baltimore, March 2016.

32. Schumaker, *Africanizing Anthropology*, 6.

33. Hawley, interview with author; and Nahlen, interview with author.

34. Penelope Phillips-Howard, interview with author.

35. Evan Mathenge, interview with author; S. Patrick Kachur, interview with author; and John Gimnig, interview with author.

36. Amos Odhacha, interview with author.

37. Elliott and Koech, *Reimagining Science*.

38. Onyango, interview with author; and George Okoth, interview with author.

39. Letter, Karen Shelley to Penelope Phillips-Howard, March 26, 1996, Randall Packard, personal papers, Baltimore, MD.

40. Phillips-Howard, interview with author; and Onyango, interview with author.

41. Kachur, interview with author.

42. Kachur, interview with author.

43. Sarah Atieno,* interview with author, Rarieda-Omiyomano (Asembo), August 18, 2015. I use pseudonyms (marked in the notes with an asterisk) for my informants who were involved in the trial as former participants and *nyamrerwa*. For more on the origins of *nyamrerwa* in Siaya, see Aellah and Okoth, "'Living honourably and independently,'" 108.

44. Atieno,* interview with author.

45. Benta Kamire, interview with author.

46. Henke, "Making a place for science."

47. Hawley, interview with author.

48. Geissler and Prince, *Land Is Dying*, 22–23. Michael Onyango also told me how people sometimes linked researchers' questionnaires to concerns about potential theft (for instance, theft of cattle following questions about how many cattle they owned).

49. Geissler and Prince, *Land Is Dying*, 300.

50. Cohen and Odhiambo, *Siaya*, 43–60. Onyango, interview with author.

51. The experiment remained internally valid since neither the intervention nor the control group seemed significantly more affected by these. Of course, critics of randomized controlled trials have argued that the internal validity of a randomized controlled trial—the

extent to which its findings support a claim about cause and effect in a specific study—is not the same as its external validity, or the ability of the findings to be generalized to other settings. Worrall, "Why there's no cause to randomize"; Cartwright, "What are randomised controlled trials good for?"; and Deaton and Cartwright, "Understanding and misunderstanding."

52. Fax, Penelope Phillips-Howard to Karen Shelley, March 1, 1996, Randall Packard, personal papers.

53. Phillips-Howard, interview with author.

54. Geissler and Molyneux, *Evidence, Ethos, and Experiment*; and Graboyes, *Experiment Must Continue*.

55. Letter, Penelope Phillips-Howard to Karen Shelley, January 26, 1996, Randall Packard, personal papers.

56. Bednet study cross-sectional survey consent form [English version], 1996, CDC Archives, Atlanta. For more on how people in this area described anemia and blood more generally, see Geissler, "'*Kachinja* are coming!'" 190–3.

57. Bednet study cross-sectional survey consent form [English version], 1996, CDC Archives.

58. Esther Adhiambo,* interview with author, Rarieda-Omiyomano, August 18, 2015.

59. Phillips-Howard, interview with author.

60. Geissler, "'*Kachinja* are coming!'" 186.

61. Jane Alaii, email communication, November 2015; Onyango, interview with author.

62. For more on the history of blood taking in medical research projects in East Africa, see White, *Speaking with Vampires*; and Graboyes, *Experiment Must Continue*, 21–50, 128–54.

63. Simon Kariuki, interview with author; and Alaii, email communication.

64. Bednet study cross-sectional survey consent form [English version], 1996, CDC Archives.

65. Kachur, interview with author.

66. Villages—the unit of analysis—were divided into groups, or clusters, of ten (forming a sector) for the trial. Phillips-Howard, interview with author.

67. Onyango, interview with author.

68. Alaii et al., "Community reactions."

69. Phillips-Howard et al., "Efficacy of permethrin-treated bed nets on child mortality," 11–12.

70. Phillips-Howard et al., "Efficacy of permethrin-treated bed nets on child mortality," 11–12.

71. Kaler, "Moral lens of population control."

72. Residents of Rarieda-Omiyomano and Nyawara (Gem), interviews with author; Alaii, email communication; and Phillips-Howard, interview with author.

73. Residents of Rarieda-Omiyomano, interviews with author; and Alaii et al., "Community reactions."

74. Alaii et al., "Factors affecting use."

75. Atieno,* interview with author.

76. Onyango, interview with author.

77. Phillips-Howard, interview with author.

78. Okoth, interview with author.

79. Phillips-Howard, interview with author.

80. Onyango, interview with author.

81. Cohen and Odhiambo, *Siaya*, 25; and Geissler and Prince, *Land Is Dying*, 125.

82. Onyango, interview with author.

83. Onyango, interview with author.

84. Okoth, interview with author.

85. Onyango, interview with author.

86. Ter Kuile, interview with author; and John Vulule, interview with author.

87. Geissler and Prince, *Land Is Dying*, 204.

88. Odhacha, interview with author.

89. Geissler and Prince, "*Life Seen*"; and McMahon et al., "'Girl with her period.'"

90. Vulule, interview with author.

91. Odhacha, interview with author.

92. Ter Kuile, interview with author.

93. Phillips-Howard et al., "Efficacy of permethrin-treated bed nets in the prevention of mortality."

94. Vulule, interview with author.

95. Mathenge, interview with author.

96. Kariuki, interview with author.

97. Geissler, "What future remains?"

98. Ter Kuile, interview with author.

99. Kamire, interview with author.

100. Phillips-Howard, interview with author; Phillips-Howard et al., "Efficacy of permethrin-treated bed nets on child mortality."

101. Email correspondence, Feiko ter Kuile and Allen Hightower, 1996, CDC Archives.

102. Ter Kuile, interview with author.

103. Phillips-Howard et al., "Efficacy of permethrin-treated bed nets in the prevention of mortality," 27.

104. Phillips-Howard et al., "Efficacy of permethrin-treated bed nets in the prevention of mortality," 27.; Wiseman et al., "Cost-effectiveness of permethrin-treated bed nets." These are rates of protective efficacy, which suggest that among 1,000 children tracked for one year, it is expected that approximately 35 additional children under the age of one and 10 additional children between the ages of one and five would survive if sleeping under an ITN regularly.

105. Hawley et al., "Community-wide effects."

106. Howard et al., "Evidence for a mass community effect."

107. Wiseman, "Cost-effectiveness of permethrin-treated bed nets."

108. Hawley et al., "Implications," 171.

109. Hawley et al., "Implications," 171. See also Prince, "Precarious projects."

110. Odhacha, interview with author.

111. Residents of Rarieda-Omiyomano and Nyawara, interviews with author.

112. Enserink, "Bed nets prove their mettle," 2271.

113. For other examples of bed net promotion in the popular press, see McNeil, "Study says combating malaria would cost little."

114. Kachur, interview with author.

115. Phillips-Howard, interview with author.

116. Arudo et al., "Comparison of government statistics."

117. Phillips-Howard et al., "Efficacy of permethrin-treated bed nets on child mortality."

118. Vulule, interview with author.

Chapter 3. The Technology of Neoliberal Policy

1. Barnaby Phillips and Gro Harlem Brundtland quoted, respectively, in Roll Back Malaria/World Health Organization (RBM/WHO), *Extract from the African Summit*, 37, 14.

2. For more on the rise of randomized controlled trial data and cost-effectiveness calculations in international health decision making during the 1980s and 1990s, see Adams, "Metrics of the global sovereign," and McMillen, "'These findings confirm conclusions.'"

3. Gaudillière et al., "Global health."

4. Packard, *History of Global Health*.

5. Grace, *African Motors*.

6. Isaacman and Isaacman, *Dams, Displacement, and Delusions*, 152.

7. For more examples of how Kenyans challenged or pursued alternative measures to state and international development efforts in the postcolonial period, see Moskowitz, *Seeing Like a Citizen*.

8. Priya Lal examined this dialectic between policy and practice in her study of *ujamaa*, the socialist nation-building initiative spearheaded by President Julius Nyerere in Tanzania from 1967 to 1975. Lal, *African Socialism*.

9. Don de Savigny, interview with author.

10. Ndege, *Health, State, and Society*, 144.

11. Letter, Hon. Mwai Kibaki to Mr. Barber Conable, World Bank Archives, Washington, DC, File 1329450.

12. Ndege, *Health, State, and Society*, 143–44.

13. B. Snow et al., "Strategic development and activity," 11.

14. Letter, Hon. Mwai Kibaki to Mr. Barber Conable, World Bank Archives, File 1329450.

15. Kenya Ministry of Health, "Kenya National Plan of Action for Malaria Control, 1992," 15, Kenya Medical Research-Centre for Global Health Research Archives, Kisumu.

16. Kenya Ministry of Health, "Kenya National Plan of Action."

17. World Health Organization, Summary Records of WHO Executive Board, Eighty-Fifth session, Geneva, 15–24 January 1990, 55.

18. World Health Organization, Summary Records, 63.

19. World Health Organization, Summary Records, 64.

20. World Health Organization, Summary Records, 65.

21. World Health Organization, Summary Records, 64.

22. Dr. Ralph Henderson, Draft Memorandum to All Regional Directors, October 1, 1990, WHO Archives, File M2-87-59, Jacket 1.

23. Henderson, Draft Memorandum.

24. Memo, Larry Saiers (DAA/AFR) from Richard Cobb (AFR/TR) at USAID Africa Bureau, August 19, 1990, "An analytic agenda: A more systematic look at malaria," WHO Archives, File M2-87-59, Jacket 1.

25. WHO, "Report of the Preparatory Meeting of the Interregional Conference on Malaria," (Brazzaville: WHO-AFRO, 1991), WHO Archives, File M2-87-59, Jacket 5.

26. Development agencies increasingly embraced "community-based" health and development projects during the 1980s and 1990s in response to what they considered the poor performance of large-scale, state-led development projects. The term "community-based" was used to describe small-scale, decentralized projects carried out and often funded by potential beneficiaries. However, the promotion of decentralized, participatory development projects in poor, rural areas has a much longer history, informed as much by anticolonial sentiments as by wealthy countries' desire to take responsibility for social service provision out of the hands of centralized state bureaucracies. For more on the history of and changes in "community-based" development, see Immerwahr, *Thinking Small*. For more on the history of self-help community development projects in Kenya, see chapter 6 of Moskowitz, *Seeing Like a Citizen*.

27. Morefield, "'More with less.'"

28. Murphy, *Economization of Life*; and McMillen, "'These findings confirm conclusions.'"

29. For more on the ideas behind the Bamako Initiative, see Keshavjee, *Blind Spot*, 72–73.

30. "Bamako Initiative" in United Nations Press Release, April 18, 1991, UN Archives, File S-1051-37-13.

31. McPake et al., "Kenyan model of the Bamako Initiative."

32. Letter, Dr. H. M. Oranga to David Evans, November 25, 1994, WHO Archives, File T22-181-19.

33. Aland Gourdin, Joint Inspection Unit, "Review of UNICEF Activities and Structures," December 1986, UN Archives, File S-1051-29-2.

34. Gourdin, "Review of UNICEF Activities."

35. UNICEF, *African Initiatives for Child Survival, Protection and Development*, 1990, UN Archives, S-1051-36-4.

36. Kiambo Njagi, interview with author.

37. "Malaria, mosquito control, and primary health care," 512. For more on UNICEF's plans to extend primary health care in Africa, see "Background release for 1988 UNICEF Executive Board Session," April 15, 1988, UN Archives, File S-1051-25-4.

38. Njagi, interview with author.

39. Lengeler, Cattani, and de Savigny, *Net Gain*, 94.

40. Letter from Dr. H. M. Oranga to David Evans, November 25, 1994, WHO Archives, File T22-181-19 (1994).

41. Lengeler, Cattani, and de Savigny, *Net Gain*, 94.

42. Snow, Mwenesi, and Rapuoda, "Malaria Situation Analysis for Kenya," 25–48.

43. Letter, Dr. H. M. Oranga to David Evans, November 25, 1994, WHO Archives, File T22-181-19.

44. Lengeler, Cattani, and de Savigny, *Net Gain*, 61, 90–110.

45. McPake et al., "Kenyan model of the Bamako Initiative," 127.

46. Segall, "Politics of primary health care"; Mansuri and Rao, "Community-based and -driven development"; and Packard, *History of Global Health*, 250.

47. Kairu, Kola, and Momanyi, "2000 KEN: Summative Evaluation of the 1994–1998 GOK/UNICEF Programme."

48. Letter, Dennis Carroll to Craig Wallace, Peter de Raadt, and Anatoli Kondrachine, August 5, 1992, WHO Archives, M2-87-59, Jacket 11.

49. Letter, Dennis Carroll to Craig Wallace, Peter de Raadt, and Anatoli Kondrachine, August 5, 1992; and "Possible answers to 10 questions during the forthcoming press conference in Amsterdam on 25 October 1992," October 1992, WHO Archives, File M2-87-59, Jacket 18.

50. In her ethnographic work on health care in Nepal, Judith Justice also pointed out that donors exert a strong influence on the policies of recipient governments. Justice, *Policies, Plans, and People*, 46.

51. David Nabarro, Speech at Amsterdam Ministerial Conference on behalf of the [UK] Overseas Development Agency, October 1992, WHO Archives, File M2-87-59, Jacket 19.

52. Packard, *History of Global Health*; and Adams, "Metrics of the global sovereign."

53. Dr. Stamps, Zimbabwe Minister's Speech at the Amsterdam Ministerial Conference, October 1992, WHO Archives, File M2-87-59, Jacket 19.

54. Memo, WR Zimbabwe to AFRO Director, November 17, 1992, WHO Archives, File M2-87-59, Jacket 19.

55. Memo, Dr. D. Barakamfitiye to WR Zimbabwe, December 10, 1992, WHO Archives, File M2-87-59, Jacket 19.

56. Hon. J. Angatia, "Preface," in Kenya Ministry of Health, "Kenya National Plan of Action."

57. Angatia, "Preface."

58. Kenya Ministry of Health, "Kenya National Plan of Action," 6.

59. Angatia, "Preface."

60. Kenya Ministry of Health, "Kenya National Plan of Action."

61. Packard and Brown, "Rethinking health, development, and malaria."

62. Kenya Ministry of Health, "Kenya National Plan of Action," 29.

63. Kenya Ministry of Health, "Kenya National Plan of Action," 41.

64. Kenya Ministry of Health, "Kenya National Plan of Action," 8; Snow, Mwenesi, and Rapuoda, "Malaria Situation Analysis," 87.

65. P. Carnevale and A. Teklehaimanot, "Planning and implementation of vector control in countries where it does not exist at present," February 1993, presented at the Study Group on the Implementation of the Global Plan of Action for Malaria Control, 1993–2000, February 8–12, 1993, WHO Archives, File M2-522-16, Folder 2.

66. Schellenberg et al., "KINET," 225.

67. Carnevale and Teklehaimanot, "Planning and implementation of vector control."

68. Carnevale and Teklehaimanot, "Planning and implementation of vector control."

69. Carnevale and Teklehaimanot, "Planning and implementation of vector control."

70. Carnevale and Teklehaimanot, "Planning and implementation of vector control."

71. Lengeler, Cattani, and de Savigny, *Net Gain*.

72. USAID, Project Paper, "Contraceptive Social Marketing II," 1988, 3, National Archives and Records Administration (NARA), College Park, MD, RG 0286 (Agency for International Development), P 560, ARC# 6171647. Due to political pushback at home and abroad, especially from Catholic groups who opposed US government support for contraception, USAID funneled money for family planning through NGOs, universities, private agencies, and international organizations rather than give aid to countries directly. The agency embraced supply-side distribution methods, which aimed to create "unmet needs" and therefore demand for previously undesired commodities simply by supplying those goods on the market. For more on the history of US aid for and approaches to family planning, see Packard, *History of Global Health*, 204–25, and Murphy, *Economization of Life*, 59–72.

73. For more on the origins of PSI, see Murphy, *Economization of Life*, 69–72.

74. De Savigny, interview with author.

75. Miller et al., "New strategy for treating nets," 161.

76. De Savigny, interview with author.

77. Lengeler, interview with author.

78. Al Sommer and other advocates for vitamin A supplementation, for example, seriously discredited results from the massive deworming and enhanced vitamin A (DEVTA) study conducted in India in the early 2000s in a *Lancet* article. Consequently, results from the DEVTA study, which showed that vitamin A supplementation had essentially no impact on child mortality, were not published until nearly ten years after the end of the study. Packard, *History of Global Health*, 323–27.

79. De Savigny, interview with author.

80. Anne Mills, interview with author.

81. Bob Snow, interview with author.

82. WHO/TDR, "Tropical Disease Research."

83. Teklehaimanot and Bosman, "Opportunities, problems and perspectives."

84. Yusuf, "Harare Declaration on Malaria Prevention," 343.

85. Yusuf, "Harare Declaration on Malaria Prevention," 345.

86. Bendahmane, "Proceedings Report," 2. Senators Patrick Leahy and Mitch McConnell pushed for increased funding to USAID for a new infectious disease strategy around 1997, citing the economic and national security threats that such diseases posed to the world and the United States (including the possibility of biological warfare simulated by the recent anthrax hoax in Washington, DC), the recent emergence of drug-resistant pathogens, and epidemic diseases such as HIV/AIDS, and the US tradition of humanitarian intervention abroad. These arguments are summarized in United States Congress, Senate, *Combatting Infectious Diseases*.

87. Christian Lengeler, interview with author.

88. Lengeler, interview with author.

89. Bendahmane, "Proceedings Report," 11.

90. Letter, Gro Harlem Brundtland to Prime Minister of Canada, Jean Chrétien, June 8, 1999, WHO Archives, File M50-372-2, Jacket 1.

91. Brundtland, Speech to the Fifty-First World Health Assembly.

92. Communiqué, Birmingham Summit (G8), May 17, 1998. Under this broad goal, G8 leaders also promoted debt relief mechanisms for these countries. Roll Back Malaria, which promised debt relief to African state leaders who joined the program, constituted one such mechanism.

93. "Contribution Arrangement between Her Majesty the Queen in Right of Canada and World Health Organization, Roll Back Malaria in Africa Phase 1," Annex A, 2002, WHO Archives, File M50-372-2, Jacket 1.

94. Brown, Cueto, and Fee, "World Health Organization."

95. Brundtland, Speech to the Fifty-First World Health Assembly.

96. RBM/WHO, "The Abuja Declaration and Plan of Action," in *Extract from the African Summit*, 6–8.

97. Brundtland, Speech to the Fifty-First World Health Assembly.

98. Nabarro and Tayler, "'Roll Back Malaria' campaign," 2067.

99. DFID, "Departmental Report 2000," 43.

100. Brundtland, Speech to the Fifty-First World Health Assembly.

101. Cochrane Reviews are systematic reviews supported by a nonprofit organization and the collaboration of researchers and medical professionals, intended to support health care decision making. These reviews were inspired by the work and ideas of the Scottish epidemiologist Archibald Cochrane, who believed that the synthesized results of randomized controlled trials could identify ineffective forms of health care, which in turn could be purged from the health system in the name of financial savings and more efficient care. Daly, *Evidence-Based Medicine*.

102. Mills, interview with author.

103. Snow, interview with author.

104. Redfield, "Bioexpectations."

105. Brian Greenwood, Progress Report and Renewal Request to TDR for "The Gambian National Impregnated Bednet Programme," June 30, 1993, WHO Archives, File M24-181-83, Jacket 2.

106. Kilama, "Roll back malaria in sub-Saharan Africa?" 1452.

107. Lengeler, "Cochrane review."

108. RBM/WHO, "The Abuja Declaration and Plan of Action," 2.

109. Goodman, Coleman, and Mills, "Cost-effectiveness of malaria control," 378.

110. Goodman, Coleman, and Mills, "Cost-effectiveness of malaria control," 383.

111. J. H. F. Remme, Fred Binka, and David Nabarro, "A Framework and Indicators for Monitoring Roll Back Malaria," 2000, WHO Archives, File M50-370-1, Jacket 3.

112. De Savigny, interview with author.

113. Pierre Carnevale, "Working Paper on effectiveness and challenges in implementing Malaria Vector Control / Personal Protection measures in the context of African Savannah," 2004, WHO Archives, File M50-87-1, Jacket 3; and Letter, Dr. Fatoumata Nafo-Traoré to Mr. Mortimore, December 23, 2003, WHO Archives, File M50-370-22, Jacket 1.

114. Roll Back Malaria, Edition "Guidelines on the Use of Insecticide Treated Mosquito Nets for the Prevention and Control of Malaria in Africa" (CTD/MAL/AFRO/97.4), March 12–13, 2001, WHO Archives, File M50-87-8.

115. Letter, David Jamieson to David Nabarro, October 7, 1999, WHO Archives, M50-370-1, Jacket 2.

116. Letter, David Jamieson to David Nabarro, October 7, 1999.

117. RBM/WHO, "The Abuja Declaration and Plan of Action," 5.

118. RBM/WHO, "The Abuja Declaration and Plan of Action," 2.

119. Packard, *Making of a Tropical Disease*, 217.

120. Snow, Mwenesi, and Rapuoda, Introduction to "Malaria Situation Analysis."

121. Snow, Mwenesi, and Rapuoda, "Malaria Situation Analysis," 55.

122. Snow, Mwenesi, and Rapuoda, "Malaria Situation Analysis," 56.

123. Snow, Mwenesi, and Rapuoda, "Malaria Situation Analysis," 56.

124. "Executive Summary" in Snow et al., "Strategic development and activity," 9.

125. Snow, interview with author.

126. Snow, interview with author.

127. Snow, interview with author.

128. Snow, Mwenesi, and Rapuoda, "Malaria Situation Analysis," 56.

129. Snow et al., "Effect of delivery mechanisms."

130. Snow et al., "Effect of delivery mechanisms," 23.

131. Snow et al., "Effect of delivery mechanisms," 23.

132. Snow, interview with author.

133. Snow et al., "Strategic development and activity," 52.

134. Kenya Division of Malaria Control, "Insecticide-Treated Nets Strategy," 11. Before state efforts to lower taxes and tariffs on bed nets, the government taxed these commodities as luxury goods. About 40% of the cost of nets was just from tax. The Kenyan government had increased taxes on "nonessential" imports, such as bed nets, substantially under structural adjustment in the 1980s as a strategy for redressing its balance of payments. Maxon and Ndege, "Economics of structural adjustment," 175–76.

135. Snow et al., "Strategic development and activity," 10.

136. United States Congress, Senate, *Combatting Infectious Diseases*, 8.

Chapter 4. The Global Health Commodity

1. Dr. Anne Peterson (USAID), Testimony before the Subcommittee on Africa Committee on International Relations House of Representatives, September 14, 2004, WHO Archives, File M50-372-2, Jacket 2.

2. Peterson, Testimony before the Subcommittee on Africa.

3. The economic and humanitarian goals of Roll Back Malaria partners, embedded in the use value of ITNs as global health commodities, entailed promoting economic stability and reducing rates of communicable disease. Achieving these aims, it was assumed, would not only benefit recipient countries but also would promote political stability, the operation of global markets, and protection of wealthy countries from disease threats. Lakoff, *Unprepared*, esp. 67–77.

4. I do not take global health commodity to be a fixed identity, but one that is historically and socially produced. Kopytoff, "Cultural biography of things"; and Prestholdt, *Domesticating the World*.

5. Also discussed in Packard, *Making of a Tropical Disease*, 225.

6. Callon, "Elements of a sociology of translation."

7. Organization Futures LLC, Report, "RBM Malaria Partnership Global Advocacy Meeting, 1–3 September 2004, World Bank Headquarters, Washington, DC," 2004, 2, WHO Archives, File M50-370-4, Jacket 2.

8. The UK Department for International Development (DFID) was by far the largest donor to Roll Back Malaria from 1998 to 2003, committing roughly US$15 million per year.

Memo, Dr. Fatoumata Nafo-Traoré to the Director of DDC/AFRO, February 25, 2005, WHO Archives, File M50-372-2, Jacket 2.

9. Packard and Brown, "Rethinking health, development, and malaria."

10. Gallup and Sachs, "Economic burden of malaria"; and Sachs and Malaney, "Economic and social burden of malaria."

11. United Nations, *Road Map*.

12. The World Bank and some wealthy donor countries, such as the United States and the United Kingdom, gravitated toward this "neoclassical economics" model, often dubbed the "Washington consensus," because they felt that state apparatuses in developing countries receiving foreign aid were bloated, inefficient, or corrupt. The structural adjustment policies of the World Bank and IMF reflected this antistate, pro-market ethos. Jomo and Fine, *New Development Economics*.

13. Gaudillière et al., "Global health," 19.

14. RBM, draft letter to Ministry of Health of recipient country, July 17, 2001, WHO Archives, File M50-372-2, Jacket 1.

15. Roger Bate, Testimony to the US House Subcommittee on Africa on "Malaria and TB in Africa," 2003, WHO Archives, File M50-372-2, Jacket 2.

16. Lengeler, Cattani, and de Savigny, *Net Gain*, 56–57.

17. Lengeler, Cattani, and de Savigny, *Net Gain*, 56–57.

18. RBM, Annex F, "Resource Mobilisation and Administration," [undated], 11, WHO Archives M50-370-1, Jacket 4 [October 2001–July 2003].

19. FY1999 World Bank DFG Grant Support to Roll Back Malaria in Africa Report, May 5, 2000, WHO Archives, M50-372-2, Jacket 1.

20. RBM, Annex F, "Resource Mobilisation and Administration," 11.

21. See, for example, Packard, *Making of a Tropical Disease*, 223–24.

22. Bob Snow, interview with author.

23. D'Alessandro et al., "Gambian National Impregnated Bed Net Programme." See also Snow et al., "Effect of delivery mechanisms."

24. Agreement for Performance of Work between WHO/RBM and Dr. Fred Binka, March 2000–May 2000, WHO Archives, File M50-87-5. While social marketing schemes showed promise in select places during the 1990s, notably in Tanzania, these schemes failed to fully overcome issues with low retreatment rates. Schellenberg et al., "Effect of large-scale social marketing."

25. RBM, "Strategic Social Mobilization/Communication to Support Scaling Up of Insecticide-Treated Net Programmes in Selected African Countries," 2003, WHO Archives, File M50-370-1, Jacket 4.

26. Jenny Hill, Jayne Miller, and Eve Worrall, Draft, "Targeting ITN Subsidies: A Framework for Programme Managers in Africa," April 14, 2005, 60, WHO Archives, File M50-370-22, Jacket 1.

27. Jo Lines, interview with author.

28. WHO/RBM, "Resource Support Network on Implementation of Bednet Programmes Including Supply of Nets and Insecticides, Report of a Meeting (Draft 3); Geneva, October 8–9, 1998," 1998, 3, WHO Archives, File M50-87-5.

29. WHO/RBM, "Strategic Social Mobilization/Communication to Support Scaling Up," 3.

30. WHO/RBM, "Strategic Social Mobilization/Communication to Support Scaling Up," 3.

31. Memo, RBM Senior Adviser Dr. Mohammadou Kabir Cham to Dr. Fatoumata Nafo-Traoré, December 12, 2005, WHO Archives, File M50-181-3, Jacket 1.

32. Memo, Dr. Fatoumata Nafo-Traoré to the Director of CPE [Control, Prevention, and Eradication] Department, March 23, 2005, WHO Archives, File M50-370-22, Jacket 1.

33. World Health Organization, *World Malaria Report 2008*, 18.

34. Including coverage of all vulnerable groups, these proportions were still less than 20% and 5%, respectively. WHO and United Nations Children's Fund, "Africa Malaria Report 2003," 8.

35. WHO and United Nations Children's Fund, "Africa Malaria Report 2003," 8.

36. Curtis et al., "Scaling-up coverage," 304.

37. Richard (Rick) Steketee, interview with author; and Penelope Phillips-Howard, interview with author.

38. Teklehaimanot, Sachs, and Curtis, "Malaria control needs mass distribution," 2146.

39. Lines et al., "Scaling up and sustaining insecticide-treated net coverage."

40. Lines, interview with author; and Anne Mills, interview with author.

41. Lines et al., "Scaling up and sustaining insecticide-treated net coverage," 466.

42. Don de Savigny, interview with author.

43. WHO/RBM, Annex A: Joint Programme Document, Project Proposal in "Intensified action to scale up insecticide treated net coverage for vulnerable groups in selected African countries," September 30, 2004, WHO Archives, M50-370-22, Jacket 1.

44. Packard, *Making of a Tropical Disease*, 231.

45. Renne, *Politics of Polio*, 44–48.

46. World Health Organization, *World Malaria Report 2008*, 19.

47. For a discussion of the mass transfer of humanitarian biomedical goods to make up for resource and governance gaps, see Lakoff, *Unprepared*, 67–77.

48. Lakoff, *Unprepared*, 289. The former head of UNAIDS, Peter Piot, acknowledged the substantial pull of HIV/AIDS in attracting global health financing even before the Global Fund officially launched. He was quoted in a June 2001 article as saying, "If various contenders get funds for non-AIDS projects, they will have AIDS activists and UNAIDS to thank." "AIDS Fund's Global Challenge," *Newsday*, June 17, 2001, A30. LSHTM Archives, London, GB 0809 PIOT/5/2/7/9 PIOT/GLOBAL FUND/ARTICLES 2001–2010.

49. Consultation draft, "An International Fund for HIV/AIDS. A concept note prepared by the UNAIDS Secretariat," March 13, 2001, LSHTM Archives, GB0809 Piot/5/2/7/3 Correspondence: Global Fund 2001–2006.

50. Senior staff of WHO, UNICEF, World Bank, and UNAIDS, Draft Note, "A Concerted Response to the Challenges for Health and Development. From July 2000 G8 Summit in Okinawa," Version 1.3, October 15, 2000; LSHTM Archives, GB0809 Piot/5/2/7/1; Piot/UN-AIDS/Global Fund/1/1; 2000.

51. Senior staff of WHO, UNICEF, World Bank, and UNAIDS, "A Concerted Response." Promoters of antipoverty measures (including control of communicable diseases in low-income countries) increasingly adopted the logic of national security after the September 11, 2001, terrorist attacks. Bernard Rivers, "The impact of the events of September 11 on private sector fundraising for global AIDS and other poverty-related issues," October 4, 2001, LSHTM Archives, GB0809 Piot/5/2/7/2 GLOBAL FUND: ESTABLISHEMENT 2001 3 OF 3.

52. UNAIDS, "Briefing Note: G8 summit 2000 July 21–23," LSHTM Archives, GB0809 Piot/5/2/7/1; Piot/UNAIDS/Global Fund/1/1; 2000.

53. The US government had privileged commodity transfer over investments in infrastructure in its development programming since the 1970s, in part to protect American manufacturers (including pharmaceutical companies). For more on this history, see Morefield, "'More with less.'"

54. "February 15–16th Follow-Up to the Ottawa Meeting. Draft," 2001, LSHTM Archives, GB0809 Piot/5/2/7/2 GLOBAL FUND: ESTABLISHMENT 2001 1of 3.

55. The United States was the single biggest donor to the Global Fund from the beginning, giving $200 million in 2002 and over $10.5 billion by 2015—more than double what any other government contributed. Associated Press, "Amid High Hopes and Frustrations, Global Fund on AIDS/TB Holds First Meeting," January 29, 2002, LSHTM Archives, GB0809 Piot/5/2/7/4 Piot/UNAIDS/GLOBAL FUND/1/3 2002 (Folder); and Packard, *History of Global Health*, 277.

56. Meeting Report, "Improving the Effectiveness of Health Investments in Developing Countries: How Is Performance-Based Funding Working?" June 2005, 2, WHO Archives, File M50-370-13, Jacket 1.

57. Letter, Carol Bellamy to Peter Piot, March 19, 2001, LSHTM Archives, GB0809 Piot/5/2/7/3 Correspondence: Global Fund 2001–2006.

58. Meeting Report, "Improving the Effectiveness of Health Investments?" 2.

59. Global Fund Working Group, "Challenges and Opportunities for the new Executive Director of the Global Fund: Seven Essential Tasks" (Washington, DC: Center for Global Development, October 26, 2006), LSHTM Archives, GB 0809 Piot/5/2/7/5 PIOT/GLOBAL FUND/REPORTS 2005–2006 1 OF 3. By contrast, the Global Fund provided 20% of all funding for HIV/AIDS and 45% for tuberculosis.

60. J. H. F. Remme, Fred Binka, and David Nabarro, "A Framework and Indicators for Monitoring Roll Back Malaria," 2000, WHO Archives, File M50-370-1, Jacket 3.

61. Dirk Mueller and Kara Hanson, commissioned by the RBM Partnership Secretariat, "Analysis of Malaria Proposals submitted to the Global Fund to fight AIDS, Tuberculosis and Malaria (GFATM), Rounds 1–4," 2005, WHO Archives, File M50-370-8, Jacket 3. In fact, analysis of Global Fund Round 1–4 proposals shows that countries submitting malaria-related applications consistently requested funds for ITNs and did so more often than any other "prevention" intervention by far.

62. Global Fund Working Group, "Challenges and Opportunities for the new Executive Director of the Global Fund."

63. Attaran et al., "WHO, the Global Fund, and medical malpractice," 238–39.

64. Attaran et al., "WHO, the Global Fund, and medical malpractice," 239.

65. Attaran et al., "WHO, the Global Fund, and medical malpractice," 238–39.

66. Global Fund Working Document: "Co-investment: a central mechanism for establishing Public Private Partnerships at country level," July 1, 2003, File M50-370-1, Jacket 1.

67. Meeting Report, "Improving the Effectiveness of Health?" 3.

68. RBM, "Update and summary of selection process for Global Fund Round 7 Support Consultant Selection Process," March 13, 2007, WHO Archives, File M50-133-9, Jacket 1; and Millington, Agboraw, and Worrall, "Role of the private sector."

69. Summary Report, "RBM Partnership Advocacy for Malaria," 2004, 1, WHO Archives, File M50-370-4, Jacket 2.

70. Working Group for Scaling-up Insecticide-treated Netting (RBM), "Scaling up Insecticide-treated Netting Programmes in Africa: Strategic Framework for Coordinated National Action," August 31, 2005, WHO Archives, File M50-370-22, Jacket 2.

71. Briefing notes for regional director for video conference on malaria (GFATM), 2003, WHO Archives, File M50-370-13, Jacket 1.

72. Randall Packard, personal communication, Baltimore, March 2016.

73. "At a Glance: The World Bank Booster Program for Malaria Control in Africa," 2006, WHO Archives, File M50-372-7, Jacket 1.

74. Adams, *Metrics*; and Packard, *History of Global Health*.

75. Birn, "Philanthrocapitalism, past and present."

76. Episcopal Relief & Development, "NetsforLife."

77. Thompson, "Greatest good."

78. Elie Hassenfeld, quoted in Thompson, "Greatest good."

79. This trend of using randomized controlled trials in development economics began in the mid-1990s and took off in the early 2000s. In 2019 Banerjee, Duflo, and Kremer jointly received the Nobel Prize in Economics for their research in this area. Duflo, Glennerster, and Kremer, "Using randomization"; and Banerjee and Duflo, *Poor Economics*.

80. The donor-financed market for ITNs was estimated to be worth US\$1 billion in 2014. Millington, Agboraw, and Worrall, "Role of the private sector," 11.

81. Shiff et al., "Annual Report."

82. Schellenberg et al., "KINET."

83. Heierli and Swiss Agency for Development and Cooperation, "How to disseminate ITNs effectively?"

84. De Savigny, interview with author.

85. Bossert and Beauvais, "Decentralization of health systems"; and Cavagnero et al., "Development assistance for health," 865.

86. Tanzania initiated targeted subsidies through vouchers while many other programs did so through the sale of subsidized nets in routine health services, for instance, at antenatal clinics.

87. Hill, Miller, and Worrall, Draft, "Targeting ITN Subsidies," 19.

88. Hill, Miller, and Worrall, Draft, "Targeting ITN Subsidies," 20.

89. De Savigny, interview with author.

90. Kweku et al., "Public-private delivery."

91. De Savigny, interview with author.

92. Curtis et al., "Scaling-up coverage."

93. Teklehaimanot, Sachs, and Curtis, "Malaria control needs mass distribution," 2146.

94. Heierli and Lengeler, "Should bednets be sold?" 14.

95. Jaime Holguin, "Sharon Stone raises \$1 million in 5 minutes."

96. Heierli and Lengeler, "Should bednets be sold?" 13.

97. Letter, Anthony Haji to Dr. Jon-Wook Lee, June 15, 2005, WHO Archives, File M50-135-2, Jacket 1.

98. Letter, Anthony Haji to Dr. Jon-Wook Lee, June 15, 2005.

99. Letter, Anthony Haji to Dr. Jon-Wook Lee, June 15, 2005.

100. Letter, Anthony Haji to Dr. Jon-Wook Lee, June 15, 2005.

101. Beisel, "Markets and mutations."

102. Mboera et al., "Mosquito net coverage," iii.

103. Mboera et al., "Mosquito net coverage," 4.

104. Mboera et al., "Mosquito net coverage," 32.

105. Winch et al., "Social and cultural factors."

106. Heierli and Lengeler, "Should bednets be sold?" 11.

107. United Republic of Tanzania, "Value Added Tax Act, 2014."

108. Millington, Agboraw, and Worrall, "Role of the private sector," 14.

109. Nkwame, "Tanzania."

110. Nkwame, "Tanzania." 10. For more on the relationship between Zambia's declining economic conditions following structural adjustment, malaria control, and malaria rates, see Packard, *Making of a Tropical Disease*, 206–16.

111. Sharp et al., "Malaria control by residual spraying."

112. Letter, Fatoumata Nafo-Traoré to Zambia's Minister of Health, July 17, 2003, WHO Archives, File M50-370-8, Jacket 1.

113. Briefing notes for regional director for video conference on malaria (GFATM), 2003. Zambian officials, however, ultimately did not sign the agreement necessary to receive the grant.

114. Chizema-Kawesha et al., "Scaling up malaria control."

115. Steketee, interview with author.

116. Steketee, interview with author.

117. Letter, (Carlos) Kent Campbell to Dr. Heymann, December 5, 2005, WHO Archives, File M50-180-1, Jacket 1.

118. Chizema-Kawesha et al., "Scaling up malaria control," 481.

119. Chizema-Kawesha et al., "Scaling up malaria control," 481.

120. Chizema-Kawesha et al., "Scaling up malaria control," 483.

121. Mukonka et al., "High burden of malaria."

122. Herdman, "Malaria Control in Zambia," 1.

123. Gates, "Malaria Forum Keynote Address."

124. Macintyre et al., "Determinants of hanging and use of ITNs," 317.

125. Macintyre et al., "Determinants of hanging and use of ITNs," 321.

126. Usher, "Key donors."

127. Masaninga et al., "Review of the malaria epidemiology."

128. Republic of Zambia Ministry of Health, "National Malaria Control Programme."

129. Packard, *History of Global Health*, 313.

Chapter 5. The Domestic Technology

1. Redfield, "Bioexpectations"; Karanja and Gasparatos, "Adoption and impacts of clean bioenergy"; and Pentecost and Cousins, "Temporary as the future."

2. Odumosu, "Making mobiles African."

3. I draw on Jeremy Prestholdt's description of domestication: the process of receiving and remaking globally circulating goods to make them usable and familiar in intimate spaces. Prestholdt, *Domesticating the World*, 8.

4. For more on the influence of African consumers on global relations, see Prestholdt, *Domesticating the World*.

5. Drasilia Anyang Atieno,* interview with author, Rarieda-Omiyomano (Asembo), August 13, 2015.

6. John Obonga,* interview with author, Nyawara (Gem), August 26, 1989.

7. Tom Ochangwa,* interview with author, Masisi (Nyamache), November 21, 2015.

8. Milo Nguge,* interview with author, Masisi, November 27, 2015.

9. Alaii et al., "Community reactions."

10. Anastasia Akinyi,* interview with author, Nyawita (Bondo), September 14, 2015.

11. Victoria Okech,* interview with author, Rarieda-Omiyomono, August 21, 2015.

12. *Wananchi* translates to "citizens" or "people of the country" in Swahili. My research assistant frequently translated the phrase "common *wananchi*" to "ordinary people," so I use that term here.

13. Paul Mbati,* interview with author, Masisi, November 27, 2015.

14. Mbati,* interview with author; National Social Marketing Centre, "PSI/Kenya insecticide-treated net."

15. National Social Marketing Centre, "PSI/Kenya insecticide-treated net."

16. National Social Marketing Centre, "PSI/Kenya insecticide-treated net."

17. National Social Marketing Centre, "PSI/Kenya insecticide-treated net."

18. Menaca et al., "Local illness concepts." For more on this issue, see also Winch et al., "Local terminology for febrile illnesses."

19. National Social Marketing Centre, "PSI/Kenya insecticide-treated net."

20. National Social Marketing Centre, "PSI/Kenya insecticide-treated net."

21. Kiambo Njagi, interview with author.

22. Eastern Africa RBM Network (EARN), Report of Eastern Africa Roll Back Malaria Annual Review and Planning Meeting, 2003, WHO Archives, File M50-370-37, Jacket 1.

23. Eastern Africa RBM Network (EARN), Report of Eastern Africa Roll Back Malaria Annual Review.

24. Population Services International, "Keeping malaria at bay."

25. Bob Snow, interview with author; and Abdisalan Noor, interview with author.

26. Central Bureau of Statistics (CBS)[Kenya], Kenya Ministry of Health (MOH), and ORC Macro, "Kenya Demographic and Health Survey 2003," 174.

27. EARN, Report of Eastern Africa Roll Back Malaria Annual Review and Planning Meeting.

28. Muyanga and Musyoka, "Household incomes and poverty dynamics."

29. Central Bureau of Statistics [Kenya], Kenya Ministry of Health, and ORC Macro "Kenya Demographic and Health Survey 2003," 172.

30. Chuma et al., "Towards achieving Abuja targets," 144.

31. Oucho, "Migration and regional development in Kenya."

32. Chuma et al., "Towards achieving Abuja targets," 146.

33. Interview subject quoted in Chuma et al., "Towards achieving Abuja targets," 146.

34. Njagi, interview with author.

35. Drasilia Anyang Atieno,* interview with author.

36. Tom Nyariki,* interview with author, Masisi, November 20, 2015.

37. Njagi, interview with author.

38. EARN, "EARN Meeting Report, Nairobi," 2005, WHO Archives, File M50-370-37, Jacket 1.

39. National Social Marketing Centre, "PSI/Kenya insecticide-treated net."

40. Kenya Division of Malaria Control, "Free mass distribution," 8.

41. Njagi, interview with author.

42. EARN, "EARN Meeting Report, Nairobi."

43. Chuma et al., "Towards achieving Abuja targets," 146.

44. National Social Marketing Centre, "PSI/Kenya insecticide-treated net."

45. Communication Initiative, "PSI/Kenya Malaria Communication Campaigns."

46. National Social Marketing Centre, "PSI/Kenya insecticide-treated net."

47. World Health Organization, "Insecticide-treated mosquito nets."

48. For more on the relationship between medical research studies and public health provision in Africa, see Geissler, *Para-States and Medical Science.*

49. *Tuafue Afya Na Maisha* is Swahili for "Let's protect health and life." Dupas, "Impact of conditional in-kind subsidies."

50. Pascaline Dupas, interview with author.

51. Dupas, "Impact of conditional in-kind subsidies."

52. The high-profile leaders of this "randomista" movement in international development, Abhijit Banerjee and Esther Duflo, even cited a paper from Dupas's and Cohen's bed net study in their book, *Poor Economics*, 49–50. The study they cited was: Cohen and Dupas, "Free distribution or cost sharing?"

53. Dupas, "Impact of conditional in-kind subsidies."

54. Dupas, interview with author.

55. Dupas, "What matters?"; and Cohen and Dupas, "Free distribution or cost-sharing?"

56. Dupas, interview with author.

57. Dupas, interview with author.

58. Lindblade et al., "Sustainability of reductions."

59. Dr. Pierre Carnevale, working paper for Study Group on Malaria Vector Control and Personal Protection in context of African Savannah, 2004, 24, WHO Archives, File M50-87-1, Jacket 3.

60. Sachs, *End of Poverty*, 228.

61. Mejía et al., "Physical condition of Olyset® nets," 159; and Sanchez et al., "African Millennium Villages."

62. Sanchez et al., "African Millennium Villages," 16777.

63. Guyatt et al., "Free bednets to pregnant women"; and Guyatt and Ochola, "Use of bednets given free."

64. Guyatt and Ochola, "Use of bednets given free."

65. Carnevale, working paper for Study Group on Malaria Vector Control and Personal Protection, 20.

66. Guyatt and Ochola, "Use of bednets given free," 1550.

67. Carnevale, working paper for Study Group on Malaria Vector Control and Personal Protection, 19.

68. Guyatt and Ochola, "Use of bednets given free."

69. Jenny Hill and Jayne Webster, "A framework of strategic options for the integrated delivery of ITNs and immunizations," 2006, 34, WHO Archives, File M50-370-22, Jacket 2.

70. Hill and Webster, "Framework of strategic options," 28.

71. Monica Atieno Odhiambo*, interview with author, Nyawita, September 16, 2015.

72. Odhiambo*, interview with author.

73. Kenya Division of Malaria Control, "Free mass distribution," 8.

74. EARN, "Sixth Annual Review and Planning Meeting for RBM in Eastern Africa," 2006, WHO Archives, File M50-370-37, Jacket 1.

75. Njagi, interview with author.

76. US Centers for Disease Control, "Progress in Measles Control."

77. Kenya Division of Malaria Control, "Free mass distribution," 8.

78. Noor et al., "Increasing coverage," 1345.

79. Kenya Division of Malaria Control, "Progress made," 9.

80. Kenya Division of Malaria Control, "Progress made," 9.

81. Kenya Division of Malaria Control, "Progress made," 9.

82. Esther Mora,* interview with author, Masisi, November 26, 2015.

83. Kopytoff, "Cultural biography of things," 75–6; and Odumosu, "Making mobiles African,"139–40.

84. Minakawa et al., "Unforeseen misuses of bed nets"; Shaw, "In Africa, anti-malaria mosquito nets go unused"; Leonard et al., "Net use, care and repair practices"; Gettleman, "Meant to keep malaria out"; and Santos et al., "'After those nets are torn.'"

85. Daniel Okal,* interview with author, Nyawita, September 14, 2015.

86. Chuma et al., "Towards achieving Abuja targets," 144.

87. Noor, interview with author.

88. Noor, interview with author.

89. Noor et al., "Increasing coverage," 1343.

90. Noor et al., "Increasing coverage," 1343.

91. Noor et al., "Increasing coverage," 1344.

92. Noor et al., "Increasing coverage," 1345.

93. Fegan et al., "Effect of expanded insecticide-treated bednet coverage," 1037.

94. Fegan et al., "Effect of expanded insecticide-treated bednet coverage," 1037.

95. Fegan et al., "Effect of expanded insecticide-treated bednet coverage," 1038.

96. WHO Media Centre, "WHO releases new guidance."

97. World Health Organization, *World Health Report 2005*; and Fee, Cueto, and Brown, *World Health Organization*, 314–15.

98. WHO Media Centre, "WHO releases new guidance."

99. WHO Media Centre, "WHO releases new guidance."

100. WHO Media Centre, "WHO releases new guidance."

101. World Health Organization, *World Malaria Report 2021*, 66, 186.

102. Janet Kimtu,* interview with author, Nyoera (Nyamache), November 7, 2015.

103. Mary Odera Ochielo,* interview with author, Nyawita, September 15, 2015.

104. For example, Druilhe, "Roll Back Malaria?"

105. WHO Global Malaria Programme, "Conditions for deployment of mosquito nets"; and Innovative Vector Control Consortium, "Dual active ingredient."

106. Okumu, "Fabric of life," 282.

107. See, for example, Leonard et al., "Net use, care and repair practices."

108. Minakawa et al., "Unforeseen misuses of bed nets"; Gettleman, "Meant to keep malaria out"; and WHO Global Malaria Control Programme, "WHO recommendations."

Conclusion. Lessons for Global Health and Malaria Control in a Precarious Age

1. World Health Organization, *World Malaria Report 2021*, xx.

2. World Health Organization, *World Malaria Report 2021*, xx.

3. Bhatt et al., "Effect of malaria control."

4. For more on the logic of humanitarian biomedicine as a response to global health crises, see Lakoff, *Unprepared*, esp. 67–77. As Lakoff explains, purveyors of humanitarian biomedicine "seek to address the failure of international development efforts to provide adequate health infrastructure to lessen the burden of treatable, but still deadly maladies in poor countries," including malaria (73).

5. Takeshita, *Global Biopolitics of the IUD*; Wallace, "Global health conflict"; and Adams, "Evidence-based global public health."

6. World Health Organization, *World Malaria Report 2021*, 26.

7. World Health Organization, *World Malaria Report 2021*, xx.

8. Paton et al., "Exposing *Anopheles* mosquitoes."

9. Lines, "Malaria nets shape up."

10. World Health Organization, *World Malaria Report 2021*, 26–27.

11. Adams, "Metrics of the global sovereign."

12. Philanthrocapitalism has generally been defined as the use of for-profit-style management and big-business-style strategies for philanthropic endeavors rather than for amassing profits. For more on philanthrocapitalism in global health, see Birn, "Philanthrocapitalism, past and present."

Bibliography

Archives Consulted

Centers for Disease Control and Prevention (CDC), Atlanta, GA.
Kenya Medical Research Institute-Centre for Global Health Research, Kisumu.
London School of Hygiene and Tropical Medicine (LSHTM) Archives, London.
National Archives and Records Administration, College Park, MD.
Papers of Randall Packard, Baltimore, MD.
United Nations (UN) Archives, New York.
Wellcome Library, London.
World Bank Archives, Washington, DC.
World Health Organization (WHO) Archives, Geneva.

Oral Histories

Beach, Raymond. Atlanta. April 1, 2015.
Binka, Fred. Telephone communication. December 16, 2015.
De Savigny, Don. Skype. July 7, 2015.
Dupas, Pascaline. Skype. August 4, 2015.
Gimnig, John. Atlanta. April 1, 2015.
Greenwood, Brian. London. June 4, 2015.
Hawley, William. Atlanta. April 2, 2015.
Kachur, S. Patrick. Atlanta. April 1, 2015.
Kamire, Benta. Kisumu. October 15, 2015.
Kariuki, Simon. Kisumu. July 24, 2015.
Lengeler, Christian. Skype. November 5, 2015.
Lindsay, Steven. Durham, UK. May 27, 2015.
Lines, Jo. London. May 28, 2015, and June 3, 2015.
Mathenge, Evan. Nairobi. August 6, 2015, and January 8, 2016.
Mills, Anne. London. June 3, 2015.
Mwambi, Dennis. Nairobi. August 6, 2015.
Nahlen, Bernard. Washington, DC. February 26, 2015.
Njagi, Kiambo. Nairobi. January 15, 2016.
Noor, Abdisalan. Nairobi. January 8, 2016.
Odhacha, Amos. Kisumu. December 1, 2015.
Okoth, George. Siaya. October 31, 2015.
Onyango, Michael. Asembo Bay. December 4, 2015.
Ouma, John. Nairobi. January 14, 2016.
Phillips-Howard, Penelope. Kisumu. October 16, 2015.
Slutsker, Lawrence. Atlanta. March 31, 2015.

Snow, Bob. Nairobi. August 6, 2015.

Spencer, Harrison. Washington, DC. February 23, 2015.

Steketee, Richard. Skype. May 13, 2015.

Ter Kuile, Feiko. Kisumu. October 12, 2015.

Vulule, John. Kisumu. January 11, 2016.

Sites of Interviews with Residents in Western Kenya

Nyamache, Gucha Division, Kisii County. November 2015.

Nyawara, Gem Central, Siaya County. August 2015.

Nyawita, Bondo, Siaya County. September 2015.

Rarieda-Omiyomano, East Asembo, Siaya County. July–August 2015.

Articles, Books, and Reports

Adams, Vincanne. "Evidence-based global public health: Subjects, profits, erasures." In Biehl and Petryna, *When People Come First*, 54–90.

Adams, Vincanne. "Metrics of the global sovereign: Numbers and stories in global health." In Adams, *Metrics*, 19–55.

Adams, Vincanne, ed. *Metrics: What Counts in Global Health*. Durham, NC: Duke University Press, 2016.

Aellah, Gemma, and Aloise Okoth. "'Living honourably and independently.'" *Etnofoor* vol. 31, no. 2 (2019): 103–20.

Alaii, Jane, et al. "Community reactions to the introduction of permethrin-treated bed nets for malaria control during a randomized controlled trial in western Kenya." *American Journal of Tropical Medicine and Hygiene* vol. 68, suppl. 4 (2003): 128–36.

Alaii, Jane, et al. "Factors affecting use of permethrin-treated bed nets during a randomized controlled trial in western Kenya." *American Journal of Tropical Medicine and Hygiene* vol. 68, suppl. 4 (2003): 137–41.

Alonso, Pedro, et al. "The accuracy of the clinical histories given by mothers of seriously ill African children." *Annals of Tropical Pediatrics* vol. 7, no. 3 (1987): 187–89.

Alonso, Pedro, et al. "The effect of insecticide-treated bed nets on mortality of Gambian Children." *Lancet* vol. 337, no. 8756 (1991): 1499–502.

Arudo, John, et al. "Comparison of government statistics and demographic surveillance to monitor mortality in children less than five years old in rural western Kenya." *American Journal of Tropical Medicine and Hygiene* vol. 68, suppl. 4 (2003): 30–37.

Attaran, Amir, et al. "WHO, the Global Fund, and medical malpractice in malaria treatment." *Lancet* vol. 363, no. 9404 (2004): 237–40.

Baird, J. Kevin. "Malaria control by commodities without practical malariology." *BMC Public Health* vol. 17, no. 1 (2017): 590–99.

Banerjee, Abhijit, and Esther Duflo. *Poor Economics: A Radical Rethinking of the Way to Fight Global Poverty*. New York: Public Affairs, 2011.

Beach, Raymond, et al. "Effectiveness of permethrin-impregnated bed nets and curtains for malaria control in a holoendemic area of western Kenya." *American Journal of Tropical Medicine and Hygiene* vol. 49, no. 3 (1993): 290–300.

Beausoleil, E.G. "A review of present antimalaria activities in Africa." *Bulletin of the WHO* vol. 62, suppl. (1984): 13–17.

Beisel, Uli. "Markets and mutations: Mosquito nets and the politics of disentanglement in global Health." *Geoforum* vol. 66 (2015): 146–55.

Bendahmane, Diane B., Rapporteur. "Proceedings Report: International Conference on Bed-nets and Other Insecticide-Treated Materials for the Prevention of Malaria, October 29–31 1997, Washington, D.C." Activity Report no. 48. Washington, DC: USAID, 1997.

Bermejo, A., and H. Veeken. "Insecticide-impregnated bed nets for malaria control: A review of the field trials." *Bulletin of the WHO* vol. 70, no. 3 (1992): 293–96.

Bhatt, S., et al. "The effect of malaria control on *Plasmodium falciparum* in Africa between 2000 and 2015." *Nature* vol. 526 (2015): 207–11.

Bhattacharya, Sanjoy. *Expunging Variola: The Control and Eradication of Smallpox in India, 1947–1977.* New Delhi: Orient Longman Private Limited, 2006.

Biehl, João, and Adriana Petryna, eds. *When People Come First: Critical Studies in Global Health.* Princeton, NJ: Princeton University Press, 2013.

Birn, Anne-Emanuelle. "Philanthrocapitalism, past and present: The Rockefeller Foundation, the Gates Foundation, and the setting(s) of the international/global health agenda." *Hypothesis* vol. 12, no. 1 (2014): 1–27.

Blagoveschensky, D., et al. "An investigation of new repellants for the protection of man against mosquito attacks." *Transactions of the Royal Society of Tropical Medicine and Hygiene* vol. 34 (1945): 147–50.

Bloland, P. B., et al. "Longitudinal cohort study of the epidemiology of malaria infections in an area of intense malaria transmission II: Descriptive epidemiology of malaria infection and disease among children." *American Journal of Tropical Medicine and Hygiene* vol. 60, no. 4 (1999): 641–48.

Bossert, Thomas, and Joel Beauvais. "Decentralization of health systems in Ghana, Zambia, Uganda and the Philippines: A comparative analysis of decision space." *Health Policy and Planning* vol. 17, no. 1 (2002): 14–31.

Bradley, Andrew, et al. "Bed-nets (mosquito-nets) and morbidity from malaria." *Lancet* vol. 328, no. 8500 (1986): 204–7.

Brandt, Allan, and Martha Gardner. "Antagonism and accommodation: Interpreting the relationship between public health and medicine in the United States during the 20th century." *American Journal of Public Health* vol. 90, no. 5 (2000): 707–15.

Brown, Theodore, Marcos Cueto, and Elizabeth Fee. "The World Health Organization and the transition from 'international' to 'global' public health." *American Journal of Public Health* vol. 96, no. 1 (2006): 62–72.

Brundtland, Gro Harlem. Speech to the Fifty-first World Health Assembly, Geneva. 13 May 1998. http://apps.who.int/gb/archive/pdf_files/WHA51/eadiv6.pdf.

Burke, Timothy. *Lifebuoy Men, Lux Women: Commodification, Consumption, and Cleanliness in Modern Zimbabwe.* Durham, NC: Duke University Press, 1996.

Callon, Michel. "Elements of a sociology of translation: Domestication of the scallops and the fishermen of St. Brieuc Bay." In John Law, ed., *Power, Action, and Belief: A New Sociology of Knowledge?* London: Routledge: 1986. 196–233.

Carpenter, Charles C. J., et al., eds. *Malaria: Obstacles and Opportunities.* Washington, DC: National Academies Press, 1991.

Cartwright, Nancy. "What are randomised controlled trials good for?" *Philosophical Studies* vol. 147, no. 1 (2010): 59–70.

Cavagnero, Eleonora, et al. "Development assistance for health: Should policy-makers worry about its macroeconomic impact?" *Bulletin of the WHO* vol. 86, no. 11 (2008): 864–70.

Central Bureau of Statistics [Kenya], Kenya Ministry of Health, and ORC Macro. "Kenya Demographic and Health Survey 2003." Calverton, MD: Central Bureau of Statistics, Ministry of Health, and ORC Macro, 2004.

Chizema-Kawesha, Elizabeth, et al. "Scaling up malaria control in Zambia: Progress and impact 2005–2008." *American Journal of Tropical Medicine and Hygiene* vol. 83, no. 3 (2010): 480–88.

Chuma, Jane, et al. "Towards achieving Abuja targets: Identifying and addressing barriers to access and use of insecticides [*sic*] treated nets among the poorest populations in Kenya." *BMC Public Health* vol. 10 (2010): 137–50.

Clark, Adele, and Joan Fujimura. "What tools? Which jobs? Why right?" In Adele Clark and Joan Fujimura, eds., *The Right Tools for the Job: At Work in Twentieth-Century Life Sciences*. Princeton, NJ: Princeton University Press, 1992. 3–44.

Cohen, David, and E. S. Odhiambo. *Siaya: The Historical Anthropology of an African Landscape*. Nairobi: Heinemann Kenya, 1989.

Cohen, Jessica, and Pascaline Dupas. "Free distribution or cost-sharing? Evidence from a randomized malaria prevention experiment." *Quarterly Journal of Economics* vol. 125, no. 1 (2010): 1–45.

Communication Initiative. "PSI/Kenya Malaria Communication Campaigns." May 4, 2012. http://www.comminit.com/early-child/content/psikenya-malaria-communication -campaigns.

Communiqué, Birmingham Summit (G8). May 17, 1998. University of Toronto Online Library, http://www.g8.utoronto.ca/summit/1998birmingham/finalcom.htm.

Cueto, Marcos. "A return to the magic bullet? Malaria and global health in the twenty-first century." In Biehl and Petryna, *When People Come First*, 30–53.

Cummiskey, Julia. "Placing Global Science in Africa: International Networks, Local Places, and Virus Research in Uganda, 1936–2012." PhD diss., Johns Hopkins University, 2017.

Curtis, Christopher, et al. "Scaling-up coverage with insecticide-treated nets against malaria in Africa: Who should pay?" *Lancet Infectious Diseases* vol. 3, no. 5 (2003): 304–7.

D'Alessandro, Umberto, et al. "The Gambian National Impregnated Bed Net Programme: Evaluation of effectiveness by means of case-control studies," *Transactions of the Royal Society of Tropical Medicine and Hygiene* vol. 91, no. 6 (1997): 638–42.

Daly, Jeanne. *Evidence-Based Medicine and the Search for a Science of Clinical Care*. Berkeley: University of California Press, 2005.

Daston, Lorraine, ed. *Biographies of Scientific Objects*. Chicago: University of Chicago Press, 2000.

Davis, Frederick Rowe. *Banned: A History of Pesticides and the Science of Toxicology*. New Haven, CT: Yale University Press, 2014.

Deaton, Angus, and Nancy Cartwright. "Understanding and misunderstanding randomized controlled trials." *Social Science & Medicine* vol. 210 (2018): 2–21.

Department for International Development. "Departmental Report 2000." London: DFID, 2000. https://assets.publishing.service.gov.uk/government/uploads/system/uploads /attachment_data/file/67962/deptreport2000.pdf. Accessed July 12, 2022.

Derriet, Frédéric, et al. "Evaluation of the efficacy of permethrin-impregnated intact and perforated mosquito nets against vectors of malaria." WHO/VBC/84.899; WHO/MAL/84.1008. WHO. 1984.

Druilhe, Pierre. "Roll Back Malaria: Technically feasible or just politically correct?" In Round Table Discussion, "Rolling back malaria: action or rhetoric?" *Bulletin of the WHO* vol. 78, no. 12 (2000): 1450–55.

Duflo, Esther, Rachel Glennerster, and Michael Kremer. "Using randomization in development economics research: A toolkit." *Handbook of Development Economics* vol. 4 (2007): 3895–62.

Dupas, Pascaline. "The impact of conditional in-kind subsidies on preventive health behaviors: Evidence from Western Kenya." Unpublished manuscript, 2005. http://web.stanford.edu/~pdupas/TAMTAMpaper07.11.05.pdf.

Dupas, Pascaline. "What matters (and what does not) in households' decision to invest in malaria prevention?" *American Economic Review* vol. 99, no. 2 (2009): 224–30.

Elliot, Danielle, and Davy Kiprotich Koech. *Reimagining Science and Statecraft in Postcolonial Kenya: Stories from an African Scientist*. London: Routledge, 2018.

Enserink, Martin. "Bed nets prove their mettle against malaria." *Science* (New Series) vol. 294, no. 5550 (2001): 2271.

Episcopal Relief & Development. "NetsforLife." 2017. http://www.episcopalrelief.org/what-we-do/our-programs/malaria. Accessed April 15, 2017.

Fairhead, James, Melissa Leach, and Mary Small. "Where techno-science meets poverty: Medical research and the economy of blood in The Gambia, West Africa." *Social Science & Medicine* vol. 63, no. 4 (2006): 1109–20.

Fee, Elizabeth, Marcos Cueto, and Theodore Brown. *The World Health Organization: A History*. Cambridge: Cambridge University Press, 2019.

Fegan, Greg, et al. "Effect of expanded insecticide-treated bednet coverage on child survival in rural Kenya: A longitudinal study." *Lancet* vol. 370, no. 9592 (2007): 1035–39.

Feierman, Steve. "When physicians meet: Local medical knowledge and global public goods." In Geissler and Molyneux, *Evidence, Ethos, and Experiment*, 171–96.

Gallup, John, and Jeffrey Sachs. "The economic burden of malaria." *American Journal of Tropical Medicine and Hygiene* vol. 64, suppl. 1 (2001): 85–96.

Gates, Bill. "Malaria Forum Keynote Address." October 17, 2007. http://www.gatesfoundation.org/ media-center/speeches/2007/10/bill-gates-malaria-forum.

Gaudillière, Jean-Paul, et al. "Global health and the new world order: Introduction." In Jean-Paul Gaudillière et al., eds., *Global Health and the New World Order: Historical and Anthropological Approaches to a Changing Regime of Governance*. Manchester: University of Manchester Press, 2020. 1–28.

Geissler, P. Wenzel. "'*Kachinja* are coming!': Encounters around medical research work in a Kenyan village." *Africa* vol. 75, no. 2 (2005): 173–202.

Geissler, P. Wenzel, ed. *Para-States and Medical Science: Making African Global Health*. Durham, NC: Duke University Press, 2015.

Geissler, P. Wenzel. "What future remains? Remembering an African place of science." In Geissler, *Para-States and Medical Science*, 1–46.

Geissler, P. Wenzel, and Catherine Molyneux, eds. *Evidence, Ethos, and Experiment: The Anthropology and History of Medical Research in Africa*. Oxford: Berghahn Books, 2011.

Geissler, P. Wenzel, and Ruth Prince. *The Land Is Dying: Contingency, Creativity and Conflict in Western Kenya*. New York: Berghahn Books, 2010.

Geissler, P. Wenzel, and Ruth Prince. "*Life Seen*: Touch and vision in the making of sex in western Kenya." *Journal of East African Studies* vol. 1, no. 1 (2007): 123–49.

Gettleman, Jeffrey. "Meant to keep malaria out, mosquito nets are used to haul fish in." *New York Times*. January 24, 2015.

Golinski, Jan. *The Experimental Self: Humphry Davy and the Making of a Man of Science*. Chicago: University of Chicago Press, 2016.

Goodman, C. A., P. G. Coleman, and A. J. Mills. "Cost-effectiveness of malaria control in sub-Saharan Africa." *Lancet* vol. 354, no. 9176 (1999): 378–85.

Graboyes, Melissa. *The Experiment Must Continue: Medical Research and Ethics in East Africa, 1940–2014*. Athens: Ohio University Press, 2015.

Graboyes, Melissa. "'The malaria imbroglio': Ethics, eradication, and endings in Pare Taveta, East Africa, 1959–1960." *International Journal of African Historical Studies* vol. 47, no. 3 (2014): 445–71.

Grace, Joshua. *African Motors: Technology, Gender, and the History of Development*. Durham, NC: Duke University Press, 2021.

Greene, Jeremy. "Making medicines essential: The emergent centrality of pharmaceuticals in global health." *BioSocieties* vol. 6, no. 1 (2011): 10–33.

Greenwood, Brian, et al. "A comparison of two drug strategies for the control of malaria within a primary health care programme in The Gambia, West Africa." *Lancet* vol. 331, no. 8595 (1988): 1121–27.

Greenwood, Brian, et al. "Mortality and morbidity from malaria among children in a rural area of The Gambia, West Africa." *Transactions of the Royal Society of Tropical Medicine and Hygiene* vol. 81, no. 3 (1987): 478–86.

Guyatt, Helen, and Sam Ochola. "Use of bednets given free to pregnant women in Kenya." *Lancet* vol. 362, no. 9395 (2003): 1549–50.

Guyatt, H. L., M. H. Gotink, S. A. Ochola, and R. W. Snow. "Free bednets to pregnant women through antenatal clinics in Kenya: A cheap, simple and equitable approach to delivery." *Tropical Medicine and International Health* vol. 7, no. 5 (2002): 409–20.

Habluetzel, A., et al. "Do insecticide-treated curtains reduce all-cause child mortality in Burkina Faso?" *Tropical Medicine and International Health* vol. 2, no. 9 (1997): 855–62.

Harper, P. A., et al. "Malaria and other insect-borne diseases in the South Pacific Campaign, 1942–1945." *American Journal of Tropical Medicine and Hygiene* vol. 27, no. 3 (1947): 1–67.

Hawley, William, et al. "Community-wide effects of permethrin-treated bed nets on child mortality and malaria morbidity in western Kenya." *American Journal of Tropical Medicine and Hygiene* vol. 68, suppl. 4 (2003): 121–27.

Hawley, William, et al. "Implications of the western Kenya permethrin-treated bed net study for policy, program implementation, and future research." *American Journal of Tropical Medicine and Hygiene* vol. 68, suppl. 4 (2003): 168–73.

Heaton, Matthew. *Black Skin, White Coats: Nigerian Psychiatrists, Decolonization, and the Globalization of Psychiatry*. Athens: Ohio University, 2013.

Heierli, Urs, and Christian Lengeler. "Should bednets be sold, or given free? The role of the private sector in malaria control." Freiburgstrasse and Basel: Swiss Agency for Development and Cooperation, and Swiss Tropical Institute, 2008.

Heierli, Urs, and Swiss Agency for Development and Cooperation. "How to disseminate ITNs effectively?" Market Approaches to Development Blog. 2008. www.poverty .ch/malaria-bednets/dissemination-strategy- bednets/26-bednets.html. Accessed April 20, 2017.

Henke, Chris. "Making a place for science: The field trial." *Social Studies of Science* vol. 30, no. 4 (2000): 483–511.

Herdman, C. "Malaria Control in Zambia (MACEPA Perspectives 1)." Seattle: PATH, July 2007. 1, http://www.path.org/publications/files/MACEPA_perspectives1.pdf.

Holguin, Jaime. "Sharon Stone raises $1 million in 5 minutes." CBS News. January 28, 2005. https://www.cbsnews.com/news/sharon-stone-raises-1m-in-5-min/.

Howard, S. C., et al. "Evidence for a mass community effect of insecticide-treated bednets on the incidence of malaria on the Kenyan coast." *Transactions of the Royal Society of Tropical Medicine and Hygiene* vol. 94, no. 4 (2000): 357–60.

Hutchinson, Lauren. "Planning National Malaria Research in Kenya 1977–2010: Space and Place in Global Biomedicine." PhD diss., London School of Hygiene and Tropical Medicine, 2017.

Immerwahr, Daniel. *Thinking Small*. Cambridge, MA: Harvard University Press, 2015.

Innovative Vector Control Consortium. "Dual active ingredient long lasting insecticidal nets (Dual AI LLIN)." 2022. https://www.ivcc.com/research-development/dual-ai-llin/. Accessed September 9, 2022.

Isaacman, Allen, and Barbara Isaacman. *Dams, Displacement, and Delusions of Development: Cahora Bassa and Its Legacies in Mozambique, 1965–2007*. Athens: Ohio University Press, 2013.

Jomo, K. S., and Ben Fine, eds. *The New Development Economics: After the Washington Consensus*. London: Zed Books, 2006.

Justice, Judith. *Policies, Plans, and People: Foreign Aid and Health Development*. Berkeley: University of California Press, 1986.

Kairu, E. E., H. O. Kola, and M. M. Momanyi. "2000 KEN: Summative Evaluation of the 1994–1998 GOK/UNICEF Programme." Nairobi: UNICEF-Kenya, 2000.

Kaler, Amy. "The moral lens of population control: Condoms and controversies in southern Malawi." *Studies in Family Planning* vol. 35, no. 2 (2004): 105–15.

Karanja, Alice, and Alexandros Gasparatos. "Adoption and impacts of clean bioenergy cookstoves in Kenya." *Renewable and Sustainable Energy Reviews* vol. 102 (2019): 285–306.

Kenya Division of Malaria Control. "Free mass distribution of 3.4 million long lasting insecticide treated nets to children under five years age, in Kenya." *Malaria Control Notice Board*, issue 1, October–December 2006.

Kenya Division of Malaria Control. "Insecticide-Treated Nets Strategy." Nairobi: Kenya Ministry of Health, February 2001.

Kenya Division of Malaria Control. "Progress made after the mass distribution of ITNs." *Malaria Control Notice Board*, issue 2, January-March 2007.

Kenya Medical Research Institute (KEMRI). "Kenya Medical Research Institute, First Report 1982." Nairobi: KEMRI, 1985.

Keshavjee, Salmaan. *Blind Spot: How Neoliberalism Infiltrated Global Health*. Berkeley: University of California Press, 2014.

Kilama, Wenceslaus. "Roll back malaria in sub-Saharan Africa?" In Round Table Discussion, "Rolling back malaria: action or rhetoric?" *Bulletin of the WHO* vol. 78, no. 12 (2000): 1452–53.

King, Nicholas. "Security, disease, commerce: Ideologies of postcolonial global health." *Social Studies of Science* vol. 32, no. 5–6 (2002): 763–89.

Kopytoff, Igor. "The cultural biography of things: Commoditization as process." In Arjun Appadurai, ed., *The Social Life of Things: Commodities in Cultural Perspective*. Cambridge: Cambridge University Press, 1986. 64–91.

Kramer, Paul. "Embedding capitalism: Political-economic history, the United States, and the world." *Journal of the Gilded Age and Progressive Era* vol. 15 (2016): 331–62.

Kweku, Margaret, et al. "Public-private delivery of insecticide-treated nets: A voucher scheme in Volta Region, Ghana." *Malaria Journal* vol. 6, no. 1 (2007): 14–23.

Lakoff, Andrew. *Unprepared: Global Health in a Time of Emergency*. Berkeley: University of California Press, 2017.

Lal, Priya. *African Socialism in Postcolonial Tanzania: Between the Village and the World*. New York: Cambridge University Press, 2015.

Lane, Richard. "Tore Godal: Quiet colossus of global health." *Lancet* vol. 394 (2019): 2142.

Langwick, Stacey. "Devils, parasites, and fierce needles: Healing and the politics of translation in southern Tanzania." *Science, Technology, and Human Values* vol. 32, no. 1 (2007): 88–117.

Lengeler, Christian. "Cochrane review: Insecticide-treated bednets and curtains for malaria control (Cochrane Review), The Cochrane Library Issue 3." Oxford: Update software, 1998.

Lengeler, Christian, Jacqueline Cattani, and Don de Savigny, eds. *Net Gain: A New Method for Preventing Malaria Deaths*. Ottawa and Geneva: International Development Research Centre (Canada) and WHO, 1996.

Leonard, Lori, et al. "Net use, care and repair practices following a universal distribution campaign in Mali." *Malaria Journal* vol. 13, no. 1 (2014): 435–42.

Lindblade, Kim, et al. "Sustainability of reductions in malaria transmission and infant mortality in western Kenya with use of insecticide-treated bednets." *Journal of the American Medical Association* vol. 291, no. 21 (2004): 2571–80.

Lindsay, S. W., et al. "Impact of permethrin-treated bednets on malaria transmission by the *Anopheles gambiae* complex in The Gambia." *Medical and Veterinary Entomology* vol. 3 (1989): 263–71.

Lindsay, S. W., and M. E. Gibson. "Bednets revisited—old idea, new angle." *Parasitology Today* vol. 4, no. 10 (1988): 270–72.

Lines, Jo. "Malaria nets shape up for resistance." *Nature Microbiology* vol. 5 (2020): 6–7.

Lines, Jo, et al. "Scaling up and sustaining insecticide-treated net coverage." *Lancet Infectious Diseases* vol. 3, no. 8 (2003): 465–66.

Lines, Jo, et al. "Tests of repellent or insecticide impregnated curtains, bednets and anklets against malaria vectors in Tanzania." No. WHO/VBC/85.920. Unpublished. WHO. 1985.

Lin, Lu Bao. "Bednets treated with pyrethroids for malaria control." In G. A. T Targett, ed., *Waiting for the Vaccine*. West Sussex: John Wiley, 1991.

MacCormack, C. P., R. W. Snow, and B. M. Greenwood. "Use of insecticide-impregnated bed nets in Gambian primary health care: economic aspects." *Bulletin of the WHO* vol. 67, no. 2 (1989): 209–14.

Macintyre, Kate, et al. "Determinants of hanging and use of ITNs in the context of near universal coverage in Zambia." *Health Policy and Planning* vol. 27, no. 4 (2012): 316–25.

"Malaria, mosquito control, and primary health care." *Lancet* vol. 331, no. 8584 (1988): 511–12.

Mansuri, Ghazala, and Vijayendra Rao. "Community-based and -driven development: A critical review." *World Bank Research Observer* vol. 19, no. 1 (2004): 1–39.

Marsh, V. M., et al. "Evaluating the community education programme of an insecticide-treated bed net trial on the Kenyan coast." *Health Policy and Planning* vol. 11, no. 3 (1996): 280–91.

Masaninga, Freddie, et al. "Review of the malaria epidemiology and trends in Zambia." *Asian Pacific Journal of Tropical Biomedicine* vol. 3, no. 2 (2013): 89–94.

Maxon, Robert, and Peter Ndege. "The economics of structural adjustment." In Bethwell A. Ogot and William Robert Ochieng', eds., *Decolonization & Independence in Kenya, 1940–93*. London: James Currey, 1995. 151–86.

Mboera, Leonard E. G., et al. "Mosquito net coverage and utilisation for malaria control in Tanzania." Dar es Salaam: National Institute for Medical Research, 2008.

McMahon, Shannon, et al. "'The girl with her period is the one to hang her head': Reflections on menstrual management among schoolgirls in rural Kenya." *BMC International Health and Human Rights* vol. 11, no. 7 (2011): 1–10.

McMillen, Christian. "'These findings confirm conclusions many arrived at by intuition or common sense': Water, quantification and cost-effectiveness at the World Bank, ca. 1960 to 1995." *Social History of Medicine* vol. 34, no. 2 (2021): 351–74.

McNeil, Donald, Jr. "Study says combating malaria would cost little." *New York Times*. April 25, 2000. A10.

McPake, B., et al. "The Kenyan model of the Bamako Initiative: Potential and limitations." *International Journal of Health Planning and Management* vol. 8, no. 2 (1993): 123–28.

Mejía, Paola, et al. "Physical condition of Olyset® nets after five years of utilization in rural western Kenya." *Malaria Journal* vol. 12, no. 1 (2013): 158–68.

Menaca, Arantza, et al. "Local illness concepts and their relevance for the prevention and control of malaria during pregnancy in Ghana, Kenya, and Malawi: Findings from a comparative qualitative study." *Malaria Journal* vol. 12, no. 1 (2013): 257–70.

Miller, J. E., et al. "A new strategy for treating nets. Part I: formulation and dosage." *Tropical Medicine and International Health* vol. 4, no. 3 (1999): 160–66.

Millington, Kerry, Efundem Agboraw, and Eve Worrall. "Role of the private sector in production and distribution of long lasting insecticide treated nets for malaria control." K4D Helpdesk Report. July 28, 2017. https://assets.publishing.service.gov.uk/media /5bad0145e5274a3dfd78dcbd/162_Role_of_the_private_sector_in_the_production _and_distribution_of_LLINs_FINAL.pdf.

Minakawa, Noboru, et al. "Unforeseen misuses of bed nets in fishing villages along Lake Victoria." *Malaria Journal* vol. 7 (2008): 165–70.

Molyneux, Louis, and G. Gramiccia. *The Garki Project*. Geneva: WHO, 1980.

Morefield, Heidi. "'More with less': Commerce, technology, and international health at USAID, 1961–1981." *Diplomatic History* vol. 43, no. 4 (2019): 618–43.

Moskowitz, Kara. *Seeing Like a Citizen: Decolonization, Development, and the Making of Kenya, 1945–1980*. Athens: Ohio University Press, 2019.

Mukonka, Victor, et al. "High burden of malaria following scale-up of control interventions in Nchelenge District, Luapula Province, Zambia." *Malaria Journal* vol. 13, no. 1 (2014): 153–58.

Murphy, Michelle. *Economization of Life*. Durham, NC: Duke University Press, 2017.

Mutinga, Mutuku, et al. "Malaria prevalence and morbidity in relation to the use of permethrin-treated wall cloths in Kenya." *East African Medical Journal* vol. 70, no. 12 (1993): 756–62.

Mutinga, Mutuku, et al. "The use of permethrin-impregnated wall cloth (mbu cloth) for control of vectors of malaria and leishmaniases in Kenya—I: Effect on mosquito populations." *International Journal of Tropical Insect Science* vol. 13, no. 2 (1992): 151–61.

Mutongi, Kenda. *Worries of the Heart: Widows, Family, and Community in Kenya*. Chicago: University of Chicago Press, 2007.

Muyanga, Milu, and Phillip Musyoka. "Household incomes and poverty dynamics in rural Kenya: A panel data analysis." African Economic Research Consortium Research Paper. November 2014. www.africaportal.org

Nabarro, David, and Elizabeth Tayler. "The 'Roll Back Malaria' campaign." *Science* vol. 280, no. 5372 (1998): 2067–68.

National Social Marketing Centre. "PSI/Kenya insecticide-treated net social marketing Programme." 2010. http://www.thensmc.com/resources/showcase/psikenya-insecticide -treated-net-social-marketing-programme. Accessed May 17, 2017.

Ndege, George. *Health, State, and Society in Kenya*. Rochester, NY: Rochester University Press, 2001.

Nevill, C. G., et al. "Insecticide-treated bednets reduce mortality and severe morbidity among children on the Kenyan coast." *Tropical Medicine and International Health* vol. 1, no. 2 (1996): 139–46.

Nkwame, Marc. "Tanzania: Textile Industry Walks into Valley of Death." *Tanzania Daily News*. June 6, 2016. http://allafrica.com/stories/201606070736.html.

Noor, Abdisalan, et al. "Increasing coverage and decreasing inequity in insecticide-treated bed net use among rural Kenyan children." *PLoS Medicine* vol. 4, no. 8 (2007): 1341–48.

Odumosu, Toluwalogo. "Making mobiles African." In Clapperton Chakanetsa Mavhunga, ed. *What Do Science, Technology, and Innovation Mean from Africa?* Cambridge, MA: MIT Press, 2017. 137–50.

Okumu, Fredros. "The fabric of life: What if mosquito nets were durable and widely available but insecticide-free?" *Malaria Journal* vol. 19, no. 1 (2020): 260–88.

Oucho, John. "Migration and regional development in Kenya." *Development* vol. 50, no. 4 (2007): 88–93.

Packard, Randall. *A History of Global Health: Interventions into the Lives of Other Peoples*. Baltimore: Johns Hopkins University Press, 2016.

Packard, Randall. *The Making of a Tropical Disease: A Short History of Malaria*. Baltimore: Johns Hopkins University Press, 2007.

Packard, Randall, and Peter Brown. "Rethinking health, development, and malaria: Historicizing a cultural model in international health." *Medical Anthropology* vol. 17, no. 3 (1997): 181–94.

Paton, Douglas, et al. "Exposing *Anopheles* mosquitoes to antimalarials blocks Plasmodium parasite transmission." *Nature* vol. 567 (2019): 239–43.

Patterson, Amy E. "Net Values: Meaning, Motivation and Measurement in the Distribution, Use and Monitoring of Bed Nets for Malaria Control in Segou, Mali." PhD diss., Emory University, 2012.

Pentecost, Michelle, and Thomas Cousins. "The temporary as the future: Ready-to-use therapeutic food and nutraceuticals in South Africa." *Anthropology Today* vol. 34, no. 4 (2018): 9–13.

Phillips-Howard, Penelope, et al. "Efficacy of permethrin-treated bed nets in the prevention of mortality in young children in an area of high perennial malaria transmission in western Kenya." *American Journal of Tropical Medicine and Hygiene* vol. 68, suppl. 4 (2003): 23–29.

Phillips-Howard, Penelope, et al. "The efficacy of permethrin-treated bed nets on child mortality and morbidity in western Kenya II. Study design and methods." *American Journal of Tropical Medicine and Hygiene* vol. 68, suppl. 4 (2003): 10–15.

Pollock, Anne. *Synthesizing Hope: Matter, Knowledge, and Place in South African Drug Discovery*. Chicago: University of Chicago Press, 2019.

Population Services International (PSI). "Keeping malaria at bay: Mosquito nets treated with insecticide are inexpensive, effective." Washington, DC: PSI, 2003.

Port, G. R., and P. F. L. Boreham. "The effect of bed nets on feeding by Anopheles gambiae Giles (Diptera: Culicidae)." *Bulletin of Entomological Research* vol. 72, no. 3 (1982): 483–88.

Prestholdt, Jeremy. *Domesticating the World: African Consumerism and the Genealogies of Globalization*. Berkeley: University of California Press, 2008.

Prince, Ruth. "Precarious projects: Conversions of (biomedical) knowledge in an East African city." *Medical Anthropology* vol. 33, no. 1 (2014): 68–83.

Ranque, Phillipe, et al. "Use of mosquito nets impregnated with deltamethrin in malaria control." Abstract of a paper presented in the Tenth Conference of Tropical Medicine and Malaria, Calgary, 1984.

Redfield, Peter. "Bioexpectations: Life technologies as humanitarian goods." *Public Culture* vol. 24, no. 1 (2012): 157–84.

Redfield, Peter. "Vital mobility and the humanitarian kit." In Andrew Lakoff and Stephen Collier, eds., *Biosecurity Interventions: Global Health and Security in Question*. New York: Columbia University Press, 2008. 147–72.

Reilly, Rick. "Nothing But Nets." *Sports Illustrated*. May 1, 2006. https://vault.si.com/vault /2006/05/01/nothing-but-nets.

Renne, Elisha. *The Politics of Polio in Northern Nigeria*. Bloomington: Indiana University Press, 2010.

Republic of Zambia Ministry of Health. "National Malaria Control Programme Strategic Plan for FY 2011–2015." Lusaka: Zambia Ministry of Health, 2011.

Roll Back Malaria/World Health Organization (RBM/WHO). "An Extract from the African Summit on Roll Back Malaria, Abuja, April 25, 2000." Geneva: WHO, 2000. http://apps.who.int/iris/handle/10665/67815.

Sachs, Jeffrey. *The End of Poverty: Economic Possibilities for Our Time*. New York: Penguin Books, 2006.

Sachs, Jeffrey, and Pia Malaney. "The economic and social burden of malaria." *Nature* vol. 415, no. 6872 (2002): 680–85.

Sanchez, Pedro, et al. "The African Millennium Villages." *Proceedings of the National Academy of Sciences of the United States of America* vol. 104, no. 43 (2007): 16775–80.

Santos, Ellen, et al. "'After those nets are torn, most people use them for other purposes': An examination of alternative net use in western Kenya." *Malaria Journal* vol. 19, no. 1 (2020): 272–82.

Schellenberg, J. R. M. A., et al. "Effect of large-scale social marketing of insecticide-treated nets on child survival in rural Tanzania." *Lancet* vol. 357, no. 9264 (2001): 1241–47.

Schellenberg, J. R. M. A., et al. "KINET: A social marketing programme of treated nets and net treatment for malaria control in Tanzania, with evaluation of child health and long-term survival." *Transactions of the Royal Society of Tropical Medicine and Hygiene* vol. 93, no. 3 (1999): 225–31.

Schumaker, Lyn. *Africanizing Anthropology: Fieldwork, Networks, and the Making of Cultural Knowledge in Central Africa*. Durham, NC: Duke University Press, 2001.

Segall, Malcolm. "The politics of primary health care." *IDS Bulletin* vol. 14, no. 4 (1983): 27–37.

Self, Lee. "Perspective piece: Controlling malaria in Western Pacific with mosquito nets treated with pyrethroids in village communities, 1979–1999." *American Journal of Tropical Medicine and Hygiene* vol. 95, no. 1 (2016): 10–14.

Sexton, John, et al. "Permethrin-impregnated curtains and bed-nets prevent malaria in western Kenya." *American Journal of Tropical Medicine and Hygiene* vol. 43, no. 1 (1990): 11–18.

Sharp, Brian, et al. "Malaria control by residual spraying in Chingola and Chililabombwe, Copperbelt Province, Zambia." *Tropical Medicine and International Health* vol. 7, no. 9 (2002): 732–36.

Shaw, Sonia. "In Africa, anti-malaria mosquito nets go unused by recipients." *Los Angeles Times*. May 2, 2010.

Shiff, Clive, et al. "Annual Report, October 1, 1990 to September 30, 1991, Bagamoyo Bednet Project, submitted to USAID." 1991. https://pdf.usaid.gov/pdf_docs/pdabp584.pdf.

Snow, Bob, et al. "Strategic development and activity for Roll Back Malaria in Kenya 1998–2000." Nairobi: Kenya Ministry of Health, March 2001.

Snow, Robert (Bob), Helima Mwenesi, and Beth Rapuoda. "Malaria Situation Analysis for Kenya." Nairobi: National Malaria Control Programme, July 1998.

Snow, R. W., et al. "The effect of delivery mechanisms on the uptake of bed net re-impregnation in Kilifi District, Kenya." *Health Policy and Planning* vol. 14, no. 1 (1999): 18–25.

Snow, R. W., et al. "How best to treat bed nets with insecticide in the field." *Transactions of the Royal Society of Tropical Medicine and Hygiene* vol. 82, no. 4 (1988): 647.

Snow, R. W., et al. "Permethrin-treated bed nets (mosquito nets) prevent malaria in Gambian children." *Transactions of the Royal Society of Tropical Medicine and Hygiene* vol. 82, no. 6 (1988): 838–42.

Snow, R.W., and K. Marsh. "Will reducing Plasmodium falciparum transmission alter malaria mortality among African children?" *Parasitology Today* vol. 11, no. 5 (1995): 188–90.

Snow, R. W., Kathryn M. Rowan, and B. M. Greenwood. "A trial of permethrin-treated bed nets in the prevention of malaria in Gambian children." *Transactions of the Royal Society of Tropical Medicine and Hygiene* vol. 81, no. 4 (1987): 563–67.

Sommer, Alfred, et al. The Aceh Study Group. "Impact of vitamin A supplementation on childhood mortality; A randomised controlled community trial." *Lancet* vol. 327, no. 8491 (1986): 1169–73.

Spencer, Harrison, Dan Kaseje, and Davy Koech. "The Kenyan Saradidi Community Malaria Project: I. Response of Plasmodium falciparum isolates to chloroquine in 1981 and 1982." *Transactions of the Royal Society of Tropical Medicine and Hygiene* vol. 77, no. 5 (1983): 689–92.

Takeshita, Chikako. *The Global Biopolitics of the IUD: How Science Constructs Contraceptive Users and Women's Bodies.* Cambridge, MA: MIT Press, 2012.

Teklehaimanot, Awash, and A. Bosman. "Opportunities, problems and perspectives for malaria control in sub-Saharan Africa." *Parassitologia* vol. 41, no. 1–3 (1999): 335–38.

Teklehaimanot, Awash, Jeffrey Sachs, and Chris Curtis. "Malaria control needs mass distribution of insecticidal bednets." *Lancet* vol. 369, no. 9580 (2007): 2143–46.

Thompson, Derek. "The greatest good." *The Atlantic.* June 15, 2015. https://www.theatlantic.com/business/archive/2015/06/what-is-the-greatest-good/395768/.

United Nations. *Road Map towards the Implementation of the United Nations Millennium Declaration: Report of the Secretary-General.* New York: United Nations, 2001.

United Nations Foundation. "NothingButNets.net." Posted on November 21, 2006. https://www.youtube.com/watch?v=guSbOPjG87A.

United Republic of Tanzania. "The Value Added Tax Act, 2014." Act Supplement no. 10. Dar es Salaam: Government Printer, 2014.United States Congress, Senate. *Combatting Infectious Diseases: Hearing before a Subcommittee of the Committee on Appropriations, Special Hearing.* 105th Congress. 1st Session, 1998.

United to Beat Malaria. "Our Impact." 2022. https://beatmalaria.org/our-impact/. Accessed June 17, 2022.

US Agency for International Development Bureau for Africa and Office for Sustainable Development. "USAID-DHHS Partnership in Health, Reviews from Selected Activities in Sub-Saharan Africa." Washington, DC: USAID, January 2002.

US Centers for Disease Control. "Progress in Measles Control—Kenya 2002–2007." *MMWR Weekly* vol. 56, no. 37 (2007): 969–72.Usher, Ann Danaiya. "Key donors to reinstate health funding to Zambia." *Lancet* vol. 386, no. 9993 (2015): 519–20.

Vargha, Dora. *Polio across the Iron Curtain: Hungary's Cold War with an Epidemic.* Cambridge: Cambridge University Press, 2018.

Wallace, Sarah. "Global health conflict: Understanding opposition to vitamin A supplementation in India." *American Journal of Public Health* vol. 102, no. 7 (2012): 1286–97.

Walsh, J., and Warren, K. "Selective primary health care: An interim strategy for disease control in developing countries." *New England Journal of Medicine* vol. 301, no. 18 (1979): 967–74.

Webb, James L. A., Jr. "The first large-scale use of synthetic insecticide for malaria control in tropical Africa: Lessons from Liberia, 1945–1962." *Journal of the History of Medicine and Allied Sciences* vol. 66, no. 3 (2011): 347–76.

Webb, James L. A., Jr. *The Long Struggle against Malaria in Tropical Africa*. Cambridge: Cambridge University Press, 2014.

Webel, Mari. *The Politics of Disease Control: Sleeping Sickness in Eastern Africa, 1890–1920*. Athens: Ohio University Press, 2019.

Weisz, George, and Noémi Tousignant. "International health research and the emergence of global health in the late twentieth century." *Bulletin of the History of Medicine* vol. 93, no. 3 (2019): 365–400.

Wenren, Wang, and Yang Henglin. *Zhongguo nüeji de fangzhi yu yanjiu* [Prevention and Treatment of Malaria in China]. Kunming: Yunnan Science and Technology Press, 2013.

White, Luise. *Speaking with Vampires: Rumor and History in Colonial Africa*. Berkeley: University of California Press, 2000.

WHO and United Nations Children's Fund. "The Africa Malaria Report 2003." Geneva: WHO, 2003.

WHO Expert Committee on Vector Biology and Control. "Integrated vector control. Seventh report of the WHO Expert Committee on Vector Biology and Control." Technical Report Series, no. 688. Geneva: WHO, 1983.

WHO Expert Committee on Vector Biology and Control. "Resistance of vectors and reservoirs of disease to pesticides: Tenth report of the WHO Expert Committee on Vector Biology and Control." Vol. 10. Geneva: WHO, 1986.

WHO Expert Committee on Vector Biology and Control. "The Use of Impregnated Bednets and Other Materials for Vector-Borne Disease Control." WHO/VBC/89.981. WHO. 1989.

WHO Global Malaria Programme. "Conditions for deployment of mosquito nets treated with a pyrethroid and piperonyl butoxide." Geneva: WHO, 2017.

WHO Global Malaria Programme. "WHO recommendations on the sound management of old long-lasting insecticidal Nets." March 2014. http://www. https://apps.who.int/iris/bitstream/handle/10665/338356/WHO-HTM-GMP-MPAC-2014.1-eng.pdf?sequence=1&isAllowed=y. Accessed May 19, 2015.

WHO Media Centre. "WHO releases new guidance on insecticide-treated mosquito nets." August 16, 2007. https://apps.who.int/mediacentre/news/releases/2007/pr43/en/index.html.

WHO Scientific Group on Vector Control in Primary Health Care. "Vector Control in Primary Health Care: Report of a WHO Scientific Group." No. 755. Geneva: World Health Organization, 1987.

WHO/TDR. "Tropical Disease Research: Progress 1995–96, 13th Programme Report for TDR." Geneva: WHO, 1997.

Whyte, Susan Reynolds, Sjaak Van der Geest, and Anita Hardon. *Social Lives of Medicines*. Cambridge: Cambridge University Press, 2002.

Winch, Peter, et al. "Local terminology for febrile illnesses in Bagamoyo District, Tanzania and its impact on the design of a community-based malaria control programme." *Social Science & Medicine* vol. 42, no. 7 (1996): 1057–67.

Winch, Peter, et al. "Social and cultural factors affecting rates of regular retreatment of mosquito nets with insecticide in Bagamoyo District, Tanzania." *Tropical Medicine and International Health* vol. 2, no. 8 (1997): 760–70.

Winslow, Forbes. *On the Preservation of Health of the Human Body and Mind*. London: Henry Renshaw, 1842.

Wiseman, Virginia, et al. "The cost-effectiveness of permethrin-treated bed nets in an area of intense malaria transmission in western Kenya." *American Journal of Tropical Medicine and Hygiene* vol. 68, suppl. 4 (2003): 161–67.

World Health Organization. "Insecticide-treated mosquito nets: a position statement." Geneva: WHO, 2007. https://files.givewell.org/files/DWDA%202009/Interventions/Nets/itnspospaperfinal.pdf.

World Health Organization. Summary Records of WHO Executive Board, Eighty-Fifth session, Geneva, 15–24 January 1990. Geneva: WHO, 1990.

World Health Organization. *The World Health Report 2005: Let Every Mother and Child Count.* Geneva: WHO, 2005.

World Health Organization. *World Malaria Report 2008.* Geneva: WHO, 2008.

World Health Organization. *World Malaria Report 2021.* Geneva: WHO, 2021.

Worrall, John. "Why there's no cause to randomize." *British Journal of the Philosophy of Science* vol. 58, no. 3 (2007): 451–88.

Yusuf, A. A., ed. "Harare Declaration on Malaria Prevention and Control in the Context of African Economic Recovery and Development." *African Yearbook of International Law* vol. 5, no. 1 (1997): 342–56.

Zu-Jie, Zhou. "The malaria situation in the People's Republic of China." *Bulletin of the WHO* vol. 59, no. 6 (1981): 931–36.

Zuzi, Li, et al. "Mosquito nets impregnated with deltamethrin against malaria vectors in China." No. WHO/VBC/87.939. Unpublished. WHO, 1987.

Index